CURING ARTHRITIS – THE DRUG-FREE WAY

MARGARET HILLS, SRN, trained at St Stephen's Hospital, London. She developed osteo and rheumatoid arthritis as a young woman, but went on to finish her nurse's training, marry, have eight children and pursue a long career as an Industrial Nurse. She developed her own method of natural treatment and, in 1982, opened a clinic for arthritics in Coventry. The clinic attracts patients from far and wide and, following on from its success, she has written this book to impart her knowledge and help arthritic sufferers everywhere.

Overcoming Common Problems Series

For a full list of titles please contact
Sheldon Press, Marylebone Road, London NW1 4DU

Beating Job Burnout
DR DONALD SCOTT

Beating the Blues
SUSAN TANNER AND JILLIAN
BALL

Being the Boss
STEPHEN FITZSIMON

Birth Over Thirty
SHEILA KITZINGER

Body Language
How to read others' thoughts by their
gestures
ALLAN PEASE

Bodypower
DR VERNON COLEMAN

Bodysense
DR VERNON COLEMAN

Calm Down
How to cope with frustration and anger
DR PAUL HAUCK

Changing Course
How to take charge of your career
SUE DYSON AND STEPHEN HOARE

Comfort for Depression
JANET HORWOOD

Complete Public Speaker
GYLES BRANDRETH

**Coping Successfully with Your Child's
Asthma**
DR PAUL CARSON

**Coping Successfully with Your Hyperactive
Child**
DR PAUL CARSON

**Coping Successfully with Your Irritable
Bowel**
ROSEMARY NICOL

Coping with Anxiety and Depression
SHIRLEY TRICKETT

Coping with Blushing
DR ROBERT EDELMANN

Coping with Cot Death
SARAH MURPHY

Coping with Depression and Elation
DR PATRICK McKEON

Coping with Stress
DR GEORGIA WITKIN-LANOIL

Coping with Suicide
DR DONALD SCOTT

Coping with Thrush
CAROLINE CLAYTON

Curing Arthritis – The Drug-Free Way
MARGARET HILLS

Curing Arthritis Diet Book
MARGARET HILLS

**Curing Coughs, Colds and Flu – The
Drug-Free Way**
MARGARET HILLS

Curing Illness – The Drug-Free Way
MARGARET HILLS

Depression
DR PAUL HAUCK

Divorce and Separation
ANGELA WILLANS

Don't Blame Me!
How to stop blaming yourself
and other people
TONY GOUGH

The Epilepsy Handbook
SHELAGH McGOVERN

**Everything You Need to Know about
Adoption**
MAGGIE JONES

**Everything You Need to Know about
Contact Lenses**
DR ROBERT YOUNGSON

**Everything You Need to Know about
Osteoporosis**
ROSEMARY NICOL

Overcoming Common Problems Series

Overcoming Common Problems Series

Hysterectomy
SUZIE HAYMAN

Jealousy
DR PAUL HAUCK

Learning from Experience
A woman's guide to getting
older without panic
PATRICIA O'BRIEN

Learning to Live with Multiple Sclerosis
DR ROBERT POVEY, ROBIN DOWIE
AND GILLIAN PRETT

Living Alone – A Woman's Guide
LIZ McNEILL TAYLOR

Living Through Personal Crisis
ANN KAISER STEARNS

Living with Grief
DR TONY LAKE

Living with High Blood Pressure
DR TOM SMITH

Loneliness
DR TONY LAKE

Making Marriage Work
DR PAUL HAUCK

Making the Most of Loving
GILL COX AND SHEILA DAINOW

Making the Most of Yourself
GILL COX AND SHEILA DAINOW

Managing Two Careers
How to survive as a working mother
PATRICIA O'BRIEN

Meeting People is Fun
How to overcome shyness
DR PHYLLIS SHAW

Menopause
RAEWYN MACKENZIE

The Nervous Person's Companion
DR KENNETH HAMBLY

Overcoming Fears and Phobias
DR TONY WHITEHEAD

Overcoming Shyness
A woman's guide
DIANNE DOUBTFIRE

Overcoming Stress
DR VERNON COLEMAN

Overcoming Tension
DR KENNETH HAMBLY

Overcoming Your Nerves
DR TONY LAKE

The Parkinson's Disease Handbook
DR RICHARD GODWIN-AUSTEN

Say When!
Everything a woman needs to know about
alcohol and drinking problems
ROSEMARY KENT

Self-Help for your Arthritis
EDNA PEMBLE

Slay Your Own Dragons
How women can overcome
self-sabotage in love and work
NANCY GOOD

Sleep Like a Dream – The Drug-Free Way
ROSEMARY NICOL

Solving your Personal Problems
PETER HONEY

A Special Child in the Family
Living with your sick or disabled child
DIANA KIMPTON

Think Your Way to Happiness
DR WINDY DRYDEN AND JACK GORDON

Trying to Have a Baby?
Overcoming infertility and child loss
MAGGIE JONES

Why Be Afraid?
How to overcome your fears
DR PAUL HAUCK

Women and Depression
A practical self-help guide
DEIDRE SANDERS

You and Your Varicose Veins
DR PATRICIA GILBERT

Your Arthritic Hip and You
GEORGE TARGET

Your Grandchild and You
ROSEMARY WELLS

Overcoming Common Problems

CURING ARTHRITIS – THE DRUG-FREE WAY

Margaret Hills, SRN

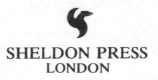

SHELDON PRESS
LONDON

First published in Great Britain in 1985 by
Sheldon Press, SPCK, Marylebone Road, London NW1 4DU

Fifteenth impression 1992

British Library Cataloguing in Publication Data

Hills, Margaret
    Curing Arthritis – the drug-free way.—
    1. Arthritis   2. Rheumatism   3. Naturopathy
    I. Title   II. Series
    616.7′2065   RC933

    ISBN 0–85969–449–6

Printed in England by Clays Ltd, St Ives plc

Contents

Dedication

This book is dedicated to my family, without whom I might have given up the fight and succumbed, in self-pity, sentencing myself to a life of excruciating pain and immobility. So, to my husband, Ivan, and our children, Michael, Christine, Graham, Sally, Clive, Peter, William and Mary, thank you.

Preface

In September, 1946, at the age of twenty-one, I started training as a nurse, at St Stephen's Hospital, Fulham Road, London. I was fun-loving and carefree, I loved to dance, cycle and swim, and my greatest ambition was to be a good nurse.

During that first year things went wonderfully well, and I began to love my chosen career. Discipline was very strict and the work was hard, but the rewards made it all worthwhile. Early in April 1947, I began to feel unwell. The doctor diagnosed acute rheumatoid arthritis and I was confined to the nurse's sick bay. Here it was discovered that I had a very enlarged heart and I was ordered complete rest, unable to wash or feed myself. A Harley Street heart specialist was consulted and he came every other day to examine my heart, whilst my progress was noted daily by the Medical Superintendent.

At this time, I was suffering extreme pain and discomfort. I was being nursed between blankets and because I could not bear the weight of the bedclothes, I had a cradle to protect my painful limbs. For four months I lay in bed, totally helpless; then, gradually, I was allowed to sit out of bed, and to wash and feed myself. The only treatment I received, apart from complete rest, was aspirin. In those days, there were none of the drugs for arthritis that are available today.

After five months, I was allowed home to convalesce. Before leaving the hospital, the Medical Superintendent came to see me. 'Now my dear,' he said, 'You have been very ill, and your heart has been badly enlarged, so I must tell you that you must never dance or cycle again. You must not run uphill, or upstairs, and you must not come back to finish your nurse's training – the work is far too taxing.

1

Also, if you ever marry, you must not have children. Last, but not least, be prepared for recurrences.'

As I walked out of the hospital gates, I thought, 'If I am to live my life like this, I may as well be dead'. I resolved there and then to do what I wanted, when I wanted, and not to tell my parents of the advice that I had been given. I had put on weight, due to swelling of the tissues caused by my enlarged heart, and also due to the inactivity of lying in bed for four months. I had gone from a trim nine stone, six pounds, to eleven stone and three pounds, and took a size seven shoe instead of size six. Nevertheless, I adopted a 'don't care' attitude, and was determined to enjoy any time that I had left. So I danced, cycled and swam at every opportunity, soon losing the excess weight that I had gained. At the end of three months, I was quite surprised to find that I was still alive.

I still desperately wanted to become a nurse, so I wrote to the Matron at St Stephen's. I asked if I might resume my training, as I was now feeling quite well. Imagine my delight when she agreed – so back I went.

By this time, I had developed osteo-arthritis and from time to time suffered great pain. However, I managed to get through my training, and on passing my finals was placed in the operating theatre as Staff Nurse. This was the hardest job in the hospital, but I loved the work, and was determined to live each day at a time. I felt that at least I had realized my first ambition – to be a fully-trained nurse.

My second ambition, to get married, was to be realized the following year, when I met my husband. I left St Stephen's, moved to Coventry, where my husband worked, and obtained a job as an Industrial Nurse. However, it was not long before we started a family, and I left work.

Unfortunately, I was now suffering from chronic osteo-arthritis, which often caused me great pain. I had always hoped that some day, somehow, it would go away, but it gradually got worse and worse. Sixteen years and six children later, I had another bout of rheumatoid arthritis, which left me totally crippled – locked in every joint.

By then, arthritic drugs had invaded the market. I went to see a well-known specialist in the treatment of arthritis, who duly prescribed a 'wonder drug'. However, when my panel doctor heard of this, he informed me that two recent deaths had been attributed to it and advised me to take it only when the pain was very bad. I was already taking twelve aspirins a day for the pain, so I tried to manage with these, as I considered them to be less dangerous, with fewer side-effects.

By now I was forced to wear a surgical collar, with splints on my deformed fingers, a surgical corset, and built-up arches for my shoes; my consultant advised me to obtain a wheelchair. My experience in hospital had made me realize that the medical profession could do nothing for my arthritis. With six young children and a husband to look after, very little money to pay for a home-help, and with myself totally crippled, unable to move without excruciating pain, the future indeed looked bleak.

I have always believed in the saying, 'The Lord helps those who help themselves', so I prayed, then set out to research a cure for myself. I got hold of all the 'natural cure' books that I could lay my hands on, and eventually hit upon the treatment that was to rid me of all signs of arthritis in just twelve months. That was twenty-two years ago, and I have since had twenty-one years of totally pain-free living.

Necessity really is the 'mother of invention', and the necessity was certainly there. My nurse's training, and the knowledge of the human body that I had acquired during that training, helped me to develop – from many combined ideas collected from the research that I had done – the treatment and diet with which I have had so much personal success over the years, and with which I am now having wider success in a busy clinic.

I hope that passing on my knowledge to readers of this

book will help to relieve some of the pain of arthritis that is so prevalent amongst young and old alike, in practically every country in the world today.

Margaret Hills, SRN

1

Arthritis – The Cause and Effects

According to the Arthritis and Rheumatism Council for Research, arthritis is Britain's most widespread disease. Before opening my clinic, I spent six years as an Industrial Nurse, gaining first-hand experience of the suffering involved, and the sheer number of man-power days lost due to this awful disease. Surprisingly, the suffering is not confined to the middle-aged and elderly. Many children and teenagers suffer from arthritis, and more and more young people are taking cortisone and various other drugs prescribed for the condition. Basically, the term 'arthritis' describes the inflammation of a joint, or joints. The chief forms are osteo-arthritis and rheumatoid arthritis, and the underlying cause of both is too much uric acid in the body.

Acid is taken in over the years in the food we eat, and the liquids we drink. If our bodies contain the required nutrients to burn up the acid that we take in, then there is no problem. Unfortunately, the food we eat today is sadly lacking in those nutrients, so we are left with the situation of an undernourished body, full of acid. This acid is carried round in the blood, until it eventually deposits itself between the joints, on the bones, or in the muscles.

When acid is deposited in the muscles, we call the effect muscular rheumatism. Both arthritis and rheumatism are extremely painful conditions. If left alone they usually get worse, reducing the patient to a morbid state of existence, where there is excrutiating pain with every movement. This was the state to which I was reduced when I was thirty-six years old. Looking back, I feel that it was all meant to be. I have yet to see a case of arthritis quite as bad as mine, but I now know that it was all brought about through years of unintentional 'wrong' eating and drinking.

I remember how I used to try to negotiate the stairs each evening, suffering unbearable pain. How I dreaded waking up each morning, manoeuvring my painful body several times before I managed to roll out of bed, crawling on all fours into a hot bath, in order to 'get started'. I can certainly sympathize with the patients at my clinic, when they burst into tears with utter, hopeless depression.

When acids collect between joints, the pain on movement can be likened to a vicious stabbing. Sometimes the joints get locked and may stiffen altogether, until there is very little movement or, indeed, none at all. In some cases, the joints make a grating sound. This is called crepitus, the unpleasant sound of the joints moving on those hard acid deposits.

Every joint in the body is covered by a membrane which secretes synovial fluid, an oily substance which enables the joints to move freely, one on the other. When acid deposits form between the joints, a wearing away of that synovial membrane is very common, due to the continuous movement on those hard surfaces. Very often, there is also a wearing away of the actual surface of the joints themselves. When this occurs, it is a situation that cannot be reversed. However, with proper diet and treatment, the acid deposits can be dissolved away, alleviating the pain and halting the condition.

The vast majority of my patients, after six weeks of treatment, report considerably less pain and a general feeling of well-being that they have not experienced for years. This is mainly due to the nutritional supplements that are part of the treatment and, I feel, only goes to show that they had previously been existing in a very much undernourished body, full of toxic acid.

In 1928, at a conference in Bath, Sir W. Farquhar Buzzard (physician to King George V), was reported to have said that the medical profession did not know the cause of rheumatism – a disease that was costing the nation £20,000,000 every year, through loss of work. To date, not very much progress has been made. They now know the cause of rheumatism and arthritis, but do not know how to treat it effectively. Patients are pumped with drugs until their long-suffering, undernourished bodies can take no more. They are then told that there is no cure, and that they must 'learn to live with it'.

Nature cure practitioners everywhere recognize rheumatism as a disease caused by faulty diet. The same applies to arthritis, although this is a more serious disease, and will take longer to correct. The medical profession today is very seriously overworked and understaffed. Doctors simply do not have the time to concentrate on each individual case, and unfortunately, the average person is largely unwilling to take the responsibility for his own health, while being quick to blame the doctor if he cannot produce an instant wonder-drug to put right the condition that has been unwittingly self-inflicted. The doctor is faced with a situation where there is a great deal of suffering borne through pain, very often hardship and frustration through loss of earning capacity, and worst of all, no hope for the future.

Recently, a girl of eighteen came to my clinic for consultation. She was an attractive girl, but her hands were deformed and she was in great pain. She told me that she was studying for her 'A' Levels, but when I asked her what she was hoping to do with her life, both she and her mother burst into tears. They told me that she had hoped to become a chemist, but since nothing could be done for her arthritis, she could not look forward to a career or marriage and, before long, would probably be confined to a wheelchair. What a sad, hopeless outlook for a young girl.

Day after day, the doctor is faced with this kind of situation, and since he has no effective 'tools' to work with, what a frustrating situation it must be for him. Doctors are very caring people – as a State Registered Nurse, I speak from experience. They have a tremendous responsibility to bear – that of their patients' health – and too often receive little gratitude for their efforts. Yet they persevere, still caring and mostly cheerful. If this book helps in any way to relieve the strain on doctors, and the suffering borne by arthritics, then it will have been well worth the effort involved.

Conditions related to arthritis

We have established, then, that rheumatism and arthritis are caused by deposits of uric acid in the body. However, the reader may not be aware that these conditions are very often connected with cataracts, catarrh, hiatus hernia, diverticulitis, gallstones, kidney stones, and a host of other ailments, directly or indirectly related to faulty diet.

Refined sugar, white bread, refined cereals, beef and pork, are widely eaten today, and all leave behind them a residue of toxic acids in the body. Modern refining techniques, and over-cooking, destroy the alkaline mineral salts essential to the neutralization of these acids which, unchecked, soon pile up in the system. First to come under attack from the acids is the mucous membrane, a continuous sheath leading from mouth to anus. The primary build-up of acid in this area can cause those conditions previously mentioned. Eventually, the acid deposits itself between the joints, on the bones and in the muscles. We are then faced with a condition which can form the basis of many diseases in the body.

The body is now unable to function normally, and various pains occur – headaches, migraine, pains in the joints and muscles, cramps, pins and needles. The spine is very often the site of arthritis, resulting in severe misalignment of the vertebrae. Every area of the body is controlled by the nerves that run down the spinal column. Vertebrae fused by deposits of acid will invariably affect the part of the body that they serve. Let us take a look at the many areas of the body which may be affected by deposits of acid in the cervical, lumbar, or dorsal vertebrae.

The cervical vertebrae
Deposits of acid in the cervical vertebrae may affect:

The blood supply to the head
The pituitary gland
The scalp
Bones of the face
The brain
Inner and middle ear
Sympathetic nervous system

The eyes/optic nerve
Auditory nerve
Sinuses
Mastoid bones
Tongue, teeth, nose and lips
Mouth and Eustachian tubes
Vocal cords

Neck glands
Pharynx
Neck muscles
Shoulders
Tonsils
Thyroid gland
Bursae in the shoulders and elbows

All this interference in the body may bring about:

headaches, nervousness, insomnia, head colds, high blood pressure, migraine, mental conditions, nervous breakdown, sleeping sickness, chronic neuralgia, tiredness, dizziness, vertigo, St Vitus's Dance, eye trouble, earache, fainting spells, neuritis, acne, pimples, eczema, hay fever, catarrh, deafness, throat conditions, quinsy, stiff neck, pain in the upper arm, thyroid conditions and certain cases of blindness.

The dorsal vertebrae
There are twelve dorsal vertebrae in the spinal column. Misalignment here may cause functional heart conditions and chest pains. Also at risk are the valves and coverings of the heart, the coronary arteries, lungs, bronchial tubes, pleura, and chest. Problems in these areas can give rise to bronchitis, pleurisy, pneumonia, shortness of breath, and pains in the lower arms and hands.

The gall bladder and common duct may be affected, leading to gallstones, jaundice and shingles. The liver and solar plexus are also dependent on this area of the spine for

9

their healthy nerve supply. Interference with the dorsal vertebrae may cause liver conditions to occur, plus anaemia, poor circulation, low blood pressure and fevers. The stomach must also be included in this section, impairment of which gives rise to indigestion, nervous stomach, heartburn and dyspepsia. The pancreas, islands of Langerhans, and the duodenum may be affected too, and interference with these may result in diabetes, ulcers, or gastritis.

Other parts of the body dependent on the proper alignment of the dorsal vertebrae, are:

Spleen	Kidneys	Fallopian tubes
Diaphragm	Urethra	Lymph glands
Adrenals	Small intestines	

Interference in these areas can cause:

hiccoughs, lowered resistance, allergies, hives, kidney trouble, hardening of the arteries, chronic tiredness, nephritis, pyelitis, skin conditions (such as acne, pimples, eczema or boils), and, in certain circumstances, sterility.

All the aforementioned ailments may be directly attributed to arthritis in the dorsal vertebrae.

Lumbar vertebrae
There are five lumbar vertebrae in the spinal column, and this is the area most commonly affected by misalignment due to arthritis.

Arthritis in the lumbar region of the spine can give rise to:

constipation, colitis, dysentery, diarrhoea, ruptures, hernias, appendicitis, cramps, difficult breathing, acidosis, varicose veins, bladder trouble, menstrual problems, bedwetting, impotency, change of life symptoms, and many knee pains.

Common complaints arising from arthritis in the lumbar vertebrae, are:

sciatica, lumbago, painful or too frequent urination, and backache.

The lower legs, ankles and feet can also be affected by lumbar misalignment, resulting in:

Poor circulation in the legs	Weak ankles and arches	Weakness in the legs
Swollen ankles	Cold feet	

The sacrum and coccyx may be affected, the former causing sacroiliac conditions and curvature of the spine, and the latter giving rise to haemorrhoids, pruritis, and pain at the end of the spine when sitting.

You will see from this long list of complaints that arthritis of the spine can set up in the body many continuous painful conditions, which make life unbearable for the long-suffering patient.

Of course, the spine is not the only place in the body subject to arthritis. It is very common in the hands, feet, shoulders and knees; in fact, any and every joint of the body is liable to come under attack from this disease. Arthritis attacks the bony structure of the body, and the reason for this is very simple to understand. We have established that arthritis is caused by a build up of acids in the body, derived from years of faulty diet. When large quantities of acid steadily build up in the system, they have to deposit themselves somewhere, and unfortunately, they have a very great affinity with the bony structure of our bodies. This affinity is with the organic lime which is a prominent constituent of bony material.

Lime is an alkaline substance. By attraction of opposites, the acids in the body are inevitably drawn to this alkaline substance, for 'mutual neutralization'. The result

11

of this process is an inflamed acid condition, which causes the joints to swell and become extremely tender and painful. Invariably, an affected joint feels stiff and becomes locked. Deformity then occurs, due to the erosive action on the bones of the acid impurities. The joint is now rendered incapable of performing its natural action. As a matter of interest, the lower parts of the body almost always seem to be the worst affected by chronic arthritis. I think this is because these lower parts bear the weight of the body. Also, the blood circulation is not as active in the lower regions.

Gout is a condition very often associated with arthritis. Gout was once considered to be a rich man's disease – due to the theory that it was caused by excessive alcohol consumption. Here again, the culprit is a surfeit of acid waste in the blood and tissues, no doubt aggravated by years of poor diet. I have often been asked if arthritis and gout are hereditary – well, of course, they can be. If an expectant mother's body is full of acid, there is a great possibility that her baby will be born with too much acid in the blood. This may give rise, very early in childhood, to digestive disorders, a tendency to colds and catarrh, bronchial troubles and, very often, infantile eczema and other skin disorders.

I have recently been alarmed by the increasing number of child sufferers from arthritis. A child is entirely dependent on its mother for a healthy start in life. If the mother is not educated as to the necessary kind of nourishing foods to eat, in order to maintain her own bodily health, there is very little hope that the developing foetus will obtain the healthy start that is its right. There is a saying: 'The hand that rocks the cradle, rules the world' – how true! The health of the nation is dependent upon mothers. Without a healthy nation, we cannot expect the output of our work force to be of the quality necessary to maintain a first-class economy.

People are generally unaware of their body's requirements, or of what nutrition is needed in order to maintain bodily health. Ironically, those with the most money seem to be those most likely to exist on a vitamin-deficient diet, often over-indulging in alcohol. One does not need to be rich to eat for health. Fresh vegetables and fruit, for example, are still relatively cheap and easy to obtain, as are cheese, chicken and fish, which provide sufficient protein for a healthy diet. Later in this book, I shall be talking in more detail about the diets necessary to arthritis-free living, with regard to both prevention and cure.

Patients often tell me that their arthritis began when they fell, broke a limb, pulled a muscle, or strained a tendon. They therefore attribute their arthritis to the injury. However, this is not directly the case, although to a person uninitiated into the cause of arthritis, it certainly may appear to be so.

When an injury occurs to any part of the body, an alkaline reaction is set up at the site of that injury. As I have already mentioned, the acids in the body are inevitably attracted to this alkaline site for mutual neutralization. The resulting effect is a 'triggering off' of a rheumatic condition, causing both pain and swelling in the affected area. If a joint is involved, decalcification may occur in the bones, giving rise to deformity and loss of power and movement. However, if a person does not have too much uric acid in the system to begin with, this situation will not arise. The natural healing power of the body will immediately come to the rescue, thereby promoting the health of the limb concerned without further complications. The reader may deduce from the foregoing statement that the cause of arthritis at the site of an injury is not due to the injury itself, but rather to the toxic state of the whole body, abused by years of faulty diet.

I am often asked if there is such a thing as 'spontaneous remission', that is, when the disease disappears for no obvious reason. I must say that I do not think there is. What may seem a natural remission to the uninitiated is, in reality, the body's own healing powers overcoming the disease, but it is my opinion that no disease will just bow out gracefully, adopting the attitude of 'O.K., you win', without a determined effort of self-help being undertaken by the sufferer.

From the foregoing chapter, it should be very obvious to the reader why no 'magic drug' has yet been found to cure or relieve arthritis. In the following chapter I shall describe the drugs which are currently available, their dangerous side-effects, and their inefficiency in the treatment and cure of arthritis.

2

Drugs and Their Side-effects

Arthritis is systemic – meaning that once it appears in any one joint there is no doubt that there are deposits of toxic acid throughout the patient's entire body. Perhaps these deposits have not, as yet, become inflamed, but sooner or later they will, reducing the sufferer to a debilitating and excrutiatingly painful state of immobility. As I have said before, there is no magic drug that will give lasting relief from arthritis, simply because the patient's body is loaded with deposits of uric acid, which must be got rid of before one can hope for any long-term success.

At present, arthritis is treated either with drugs, pain-killers, or surgery. When a joint becomes inflamed, the doctor will usually prescribe an anti-inflammatory drug which, as a rule, will suppress the inflammation, halt the condition, and thus bring relief – but only temporarily. Before long, the inflammation will rear its ugly head again, causing more pain than ever. A stronger and more power-ful drug will then be administered, and the story repeats itself until invariably the joint, or joints concerned, be-come so tender and stiff that the slightest movement brings intense pain. The patient eventually becomes immune to the drugs administered and the only course left open to the frustrated doctor is to suggest a new hip joint, knee joints or whatever.

The unfortunate patient is then directed to the rheuma-tologist who will put him on the waiting list. Many of my patients have been on the waiting list for at least two years for an operation of this kind. Whilst on the waiting list, they are pumped with anti-rheumatic drugs which set up day by day side-effects in their bodies, that invariably lead to some form of 'doctor-induced' disease. Hospitals today are full of patients who have fallen victim to the side-effects of drugs and antibiotics. Drugs drain the body of nutrition, especially iron, and the vast majority of patients on drugs are anaemic. Many are aware of the dangers of such treatment and are very loathe to accept any form of drug. Unfortunately, when pain becomes intense – as it does with arthritis – the sufferer feels such a burden to himself, and to others, that he has no alternative but to submit to a course of treatment which may, but very often does not, relieve his suffering.

Of course, a new joint will not remove the acids that are causing the trouble. Sooner or later, another hip or knee joint, or perhaps both, will be necessary. The saga starts all over again until eventually the long-suffering patient is reduced to a state of depression and hopelessness.

According to Baillière's Nurses' Dictionary, the word 'drug' means 'any substance used as a medicine' and if we think of them in that light then of course there is no getting away from the fact that they are very useful substances indeed; and have a definite place in medicine today. When drugs are taken repeatedly, a lot of patients become dependent on them and are unable to do without them either emotionally or physically. Then this is called drug addiction and the majority of people today are well aware of the sad state of helplessness that is the result of such dependence.

Most patients that attend my clinic do so with a burning desire to be able to function without their drugs. They have come to realize how dependent on them they are becoming and they also realize that the prolonged consumption of them are having very undesirable side-effects.

One of the most common treatments for arthritis – aspirin – was introduced in 1899. Aspirin is a derivative of salicylic acid and although it is considered one of the least toxic of the drugs it can be dangerous to some people. Every person's make-up is different and the human body is a very complex machine. 'One man's meat is another man's poison' and what suits one person may be very damaging to

16

another. Fortunately, I was able to tolerate the twelve aspirins a day that I was taking without experiencing any side-effects but to another that dosage, or even much less, could cause vomiting, headaches or high temperature. Aspirin can also give rise to deafness and noises in the ear and it is widely known that this drug can cause bleeding of the stomach, possibly even resulting in ulceration. This in turn can lead to anaemia due to the constant blood loss. In fact, aspirin can cause severe irritation of the whole alimentary tract from stomach to anus.

Various drugs are used in the primary treatment of arthritis – these include Feldene, Brufen and Naprosyn, also Indocid. Some patients report to me that from the time they started to take some of these drugs they felt ill with various symptoms such as headache, nausea, vomiting, unpleasant noises in the ears, etc. Others say these drugs gave a lot of relief to begin with but very soon the pain became so bad that their doctor had to put them on the stronger drugs, such as gold and cortisone – amongst a lot of others.

Doctors are well aware of the side-effects of the drugs they prescribe, but can do little about it. Invariably, the patient is unwilling to help himself. Drugs are far too easily obtained. The line of least resistance and effort is often preferred to a project of self help which merely involves a little effort and the planning of a correct diet.

Prevention is far better than cure and I feel I must emphasize how invaluable a good nutritional education would be to both boys and girls during their last years at school. I mention boys because a vast number of men today live by themselves, either as divorcees, widowers or bachelors. The majority have little, if any, idea of how to look after their bodies by eating the correct foods necessary to healthy living. After all, the body is the second most special possession we have in this world – the soul being the first.

A recent report made by the Royal College of Physicians blamed excessive prescribing, inadequate instruction on dosage, and the hoarding of drugs by patients, on the fact that thousands of elderly people in Britain suffer adverse drug reactions. This report urges doctors to stop all unnecessary medication, otherwise they feared that polypharmacy – the prescribing of multiple drugs – would continue unchecked. A working party, led by former College President, Sir Douglas Black, reported that adverse drug reactions were more common in older people. This, they said, was due both to their greater susceptibility to harmful side-effects, and to the greater amount of medication prescribed for them. As the elderly are more commonly afflicted by arthritis, and the majority of them are on drugs of one form or another then, of course, the foregoing comments apply in large measure. In my opinion, some drugs made for the treatment of arthritis are among the most dangerous drugs made, and when taken over a long period of time they can create the most undesirable side-effects.

In this chapter I have briefly touched on some side-effects that may be caused by some anti-arthritic drugs in use today. In recent months quite a number of drugs have been banned from the market because of the adverse effects they were causing. This is a very good thing and it is my firm belief that it is the cause of this disease we should turn our thoughts to; this might involve a widespread education of the public on how to treat themselves the 'natural' way.

In the following chapter, I will tell you how to remove the toxic acids from the body that are causing your arthritis and enlarge upon the reasons for adopting the 'natural' method of treatment.

3

The Treatment of Arthritis by Natural Means

Arthritis is, purely and simply, a disease of dietetic origin. By recognizing this, and treating it accordingly, I have had the most remarkable and gratifying results. I was able to rescue myself from a state of hopeless incapacity and pain, to achieve an excellent state of health, that I had not known for years. I was able to raise eight children, foster another, and eventually take a refresher course in nursing. Although I had been away from nursing for thirty years, I found that I had both the strength and the mental ability to 'pick up the threads' and renew my career. Following my recovery, I continued to work full-time as an Industrial Nurse, until two years ago, when I decided to set up a clinic for arthritics at my home in Coventry. The results that I have experienced since opening the clinic have been most encouraging and have far exceeded my expectations.

We have established that arthritis is caused by an excess of uric acid in the body, and that this imbalance is created by a lack of the required nutrients necessary to the neutralization of the acid we absorb from our daily diet. The quality of food available today often leaves much to be desired. Many of the nutrients which should be supplied in our food are destroyed by the addition of chemicals and pesticides. To the farmer, a greater yield is the most important factor, but unfortunately, this can only result in a sacrifice of quality and the supply of organically grown fruit and vegetables is extremely limited. This limitation makes it very necessary for us to take food supplementation, in the form of vitamins, minerals and proteins. This does not apply only to arthritics, but also to the very young, schoolchildren, adolescents, expectant mothers, nursing mothers, sportsmen, businessmen, and of course, the

19

elderly. Having firmly established the cause of arthritis, let us now turn our thoughts to the successful treatment and elimination of this disease.

I believe that there is only one sensible way to relieve, and possibly cure, arthritis:

1 The patient must adopt a method of treatment that will eliminate toxic acids from the body.
2 The patient must adhere to an acid-free diet, in order to prevent any further intake of acid.
3 The patient must restore nutrients necessary to the 'burning up' of acids in the body.

In the following pages, I will detail, and explain, the regime that I adopted, after extensive research into the natural treatment of arthritis. Having been trained in conventional medicine, based on treatments by drugs such as antibiotics, it was with rather a negative attitude that I approached the 'natural cure' method. However, I knew that I had nothing to lose by it and thought that even if it did me no good, at least it could do me no harm.

Before starting the treatment, I discarded the splints from my painful, swollen hands, and threw away the collar that was gradually locking my neck. I took off my surgical corset, and removed the built-up arches from my shoes. I was then ready to work on removing the uric acid, and all signs of arthritis, from my body.

First, and most important of all, I developed a positive attitude. Remember, good health must be earned. In your fight for health, keep cheerful and optimistic. The correct mental attitude is a fundamental necessity if you are to have any chance of success. In disease of any nature, the nervous system suffers traumatically and a direct result of this is depression, fear and anxiety. When one develops a hopeful, optimistic and forward-looking attitude, one paves the way for greater success. Think the following: 'Disease has no part in my life, and I am going to get better.' So thinking, I faced each day with renewed energy. I pictured myself full of radiant health and vitality and convinced myself that each day brought me one step nearer to my goal.

Having developed a positive frame of mind, I turned my attention to the removal of the toxic acids from my body. The 'prescription' that I adopted, was as follows:

1 On arising, I dissolved one teaspoon of clear honey in a tumbler of hot water, and added to this one desert-spoon of cider vinegar. I took this mixture three times a day.
2 I took one teaspoon of black molasses three times daily.
3 I took an Epsom salts bath three times per week.
4 I took a full range of the best quality vitamins, minerals and proteins each day, in order to replace in my body the nutrition that had become so depleted. This was also to help in the burning up of the acids that had invaded my body and caused such havoc.
5 I exercised my joints gently. Every book that I had read advocated the benefits of walking in the fresh air. However, I could not walk, so I had to make do with gentle, indoor exercise, but I always ensured that my room was well-ventilated.

I hoped that this regime would remove those toxic acids that were causing my trouble. I was, nevertheless, amazed when after only two weeks on this treatment, I definitely began to feel better. I had more strength, suffered less depression, and was certainly sleeping more easily.

A month went by, and the ease with which I moved my fingers became more noticeable. Of course, I had my bad days, but I was not worried. The natural cure books had told me to expect this, as it results from the body's attempt to 'throw off' the acids. From time to time, while following the treatment, the patient may find that his joints become inflamed and painful. This does not last for very long, and when one knows what to expect it is so much easier to weather the storm. I consoled myself with the thought that tomorrow I would feel better, and that gradually the pain would go away, never to return. A hopeful attitude does much more to alleviate pain than does any drug. Each week brought fresh improvement and the joy in my heart when I managed to walk from the lounge to the kitchen was immeasurable. I knew then that I was getting better. The improvement quickened, so I persevered with the treatment. By the end of twelve months, I had changed from being nervous, irritable, and depressed to being a calm, joyful, agile and healthy person. I was ready, and willing, to resume my place as a wife and mother, full of renewed strength and vigour and more anxious to please and care for my family than ever before. I was so grateful to the Lord, for giving me the strength and encouragement to explore all avenues, in an effort to help myself.

I have kept myself very busy through the ensuing years, and as a result, have made many social contacts. I have tried never to miss an opportunity to spread the news to suffering arthritics, many of whom have since had amazing results with this natural method of treatment. I have found that it always pays dividends to explain to my patients why they should do what I ask them to. It usually takes about one-and-a-half hours to explain in detail the reasons why they should take cider vinegar, honey, and molasses, and the benefits to be gained from Epsom salts baths. I also explain the necessity of an acid-free diet, and describe which foods to avoid. Last, but by no means least, I explain the very important part played in the treatment by the wholefood nutrition that I prescribe.

The components of a natural cure

Cider vinegar
This excellent product is made from mature cider apples

and is a combination of minerals, organic matter, and acetic acid. In order to be fit, we must have enough sleep and exercise and, of course, a well-balanced diet. I have used cider vinegar for the past twenty-two years, and must say that I believe it has kept me free of arthritis. I think this is largely due to the fact that cider vinegar regulates the body's metabolism, through the quantities of minerals that it contains.

The hard acid deposits connected with arthritis are very similar in substance to the shell of an egg. Cider vinegar has the power to dissolve those acid deposits so they pass out naturally, via the kidneys. The reader can carry out an experiment to show how this works. Place an egg, complete with shell, in a jar or glass. Cover the egg with 'neat' cider vinegar and in two days the shell will have completely dissolved, leaving the egg intact. Similarly, when cider vinegar saturates the bloodstream, it gets between the joints, dissolving the acid deposits and passing them away. Cider vinegar contains malic acid. This should not be confused with the harmful uric acids which have collected between the joints, on the bones, or in the muscles, causing arthritis.

One has to remember that the longer one has had arthritis, the longer it will be before any noticeable results are obtained. I suffered from arthritis for sixteen years, and after one month on the treatment, could see only a slight improvement. I could so easily have given up, but knew that if this treatment did not work I had very little hope of achieving any cure at all. I persevered, and within twelve months had rid myself of every sign of arthritis.

Arthritics are often overweight, due to the inactivity forced upon them. Their joints are so painful on movement that the natural reaction is to minimize the pain by keeping still. Arthritics also tend to eat convenience foods, which require little effort in their preparation. Thus they survive on a diet high in calories, which only adds to their weight problem, making them less and less mobile. Cider vinegar is a natural diuretic, and thus acts to some extent as a slimming agent. Most of my patients return after six weeks, absolutely thrilled because they have managed to lose weight without any effort. As a result, they feel better in themselves, and this gives them fresh hope for the future.

As I have said, for the first few weeks on the treatment, patients may experience pain in places they have not known it before. The pain is not stronger than before, but rather than being confined to the joints already involved, it now appears to be all over the body. If one gives this a little thought, one can understand the reason why. The patient's blood has been saturated with cider vinegar, which has set to work on all those acid deposits, churning them up, and dissolving them away. This process will inevitably cause some pain and the patient may be forgiven for thinking that the treatment is doing more harm than good. Unfortunately, some patients are tempted to give up at this early stage, thereby losing the value of the treatment, just as it has begun to take effect. This is, indeed, a pity. When the sufferer experiences this reaction, he should think: 'It is the treatment working for me; in a week or two, the pain will pass and I will get better.'

When a patient has been affected with arthritis for some considerable time, continuous movement of the joints on those hard acid deposits often causes a wearing away of the actual surface of the joints. This is a situation that cannot be reversed, but it is possible to halt the condition and lessen the pain. This in itself is well worth striving for.

'Wear and tear' is a very general term used by the medical profession, as is 'crumbling of the joints', and 'premature ageing of the bones'. I have found that most patients who come to my clinic attach tremendous importance to each word that falls from the doctor's lips and as a result often take on an attitude of hopelessness that is not easy to overcome. 'You have arthritis, and must learn to live with it' is a very common statement in the doctor's surgery. In the majority of cases, when a patient asks his doctor if his condition has anything to do with diet, the reply is usually 'no'. I do appreciate the strain that doctors are under, but I believe that the condition has everything to do with diet, and can be simply treated with an acid-free diet. After all, 'you are what you eat'. If a plant receives the wrong food, it will wither and die. As with other living things, our whole well-being hinges on diet.

Many arthritics also suffer from high blood pressure, angina, or some form of circulatory disease. The taking of cider vinegar can be most beneficial in this case, as it is known to be a 'blood normalizer'. If the blood pressure is too high, cider vinegar will help bring it down to normal, and if too low, it will raise it accordingly.

Ridges sometimes appear on the nails, due to a lack of calcium salts in the tissues. This deficiency can also affect the bones, teeth and hair. Cider vinegar can help this condition enormously, as it encourages the body to make more effective use of the calcium derived from food. Amongst other things, a lack of calcium in the tissues, will result in thin and brittle nails, dull hair, tooth decay, and brittle bones. Cramps and pins and needles are also closely associated with calcium deficiency. Cider vinegar, by assisting in the absorption of calcium, can play a large part in the correction of these abnormalities.

It should be noted that you can expect to urinate more frequently while taking cider vinegar, due to the diuretic effect it has on the body. For the reader who does not suffer from arthritis but would like to avoid it, two teaspoons of cider vinegar taken three times daily will, I believe, act as a preventive measure.

It should now be clear to the reader that cider vinegar is a very valuable commodity in the treatment of arthritis. After six weeks of taking cider vinegar, people usually report a transformation in their skin, hair and nails, leading their friends to ask what it is they are doing, as they are looking so much better. The benefits of taking cider vinegar are endless, but I hope that I have sufficiently evaluated its use in the relief of arthritis and associated ailments. As a point of interest, I highly recommend the use of 'Aspalls' cider vinegar, as it is made from organically grown apples.

Honey

Honey – as we all know – comes from bees, and is produced to a larger or smaller degree in every country in the world. The two predominant types of sugar present in honey are fructose and glucose. These sugars are 'pre-digested' and can be used immediately by the body, to produce 'instant energy'. When ordinary sugar is taken into the body, it cannot be used immediately, due to the delay while digestive processes act.

Honey is packed with natural vitamins, minerals and trace elements. Among other, lesser ingredients, honey contains:

proteins	magnesium	phosphorus
calcium	allumen	pollen
copper	acids and amino acids	sodium
silica	chlorine	manganese
iron	potassium	nitrogen
lime	sulphur	dextrine

The composition of honey is affected by the types of flowers and plants from which the nectar is collected and also by the nature of the soil wherein the plants grow. The time of year and prevailing weather conditions at time of collection can also affect its composition. The type of flower or plant from which the nectar is taken also greatly influences the flavour of honey and its colour.

Darker honeys contain much more iron than light-coloured honey. I have found, in treating arthritics, that the vast majority are suffering from acute iron deficiency. Many have been taking drugs which have drained the body of iron. Lack of iron in the body can lead to all kinds of blood disorders, anaemia especially. This makes the patient feel tired and listless; a marked dullness of the eyes and lifeless hair are very common signs. As the patient feels 'drained', the most sensible course of action is to introduce a good, organic source of iron to promote instant energy. Honey is such a source.

Most of the 'B complex' range of vitamins can be found in honey, and it is these that feed the nerves. Most arthritics are in a highly nervous state. They feel pain vary acutely, have sleepless nights, and become very depressed. The depression is caused firstly by the stress of the complaint, and secondly by the utter hopelessness the patients feel, when told that they must 'learn to live with it'. Honey is a most beneficial food for the tired, nervous, and highly-strung arthritis sufferer. Most arthritics, especially the advanced cases, have sleepless nights when they are racked with pain. Many pace the floor for hours during the night, suffering either from cramp or pins and needles or both. Patients have told me that they wake in the morning wishing they did not have to live through another day. This attitude of mind also brings great stress to the patients' family.

As a rule, if the patient is not overweight, I recommend the taking of honey in large amounts, usually one dessertspoon to be taken three times daily. Very often, during the first week of treatment, patients experience a sense of calm that they have not known for years. This, in itself, is wonderful, and patients settle down to their prescribed regime full of hope for a future with less, or even no pain.

Obviously some patients take longer than others to show signs of improvement, but I have never yet heard it said that the treatment has not done any good.

Honeys containing a lot of pollen are very rich in vitamin C. This is an extremely important vitamin that we need daily but, unfortunately, it cannot be stored by the body. As a rule, we depend on fruit and vegetables for our vitamin C intake, but owing to its instability, this vitamin can be easily lost or reduced during preparation and cooking. For example, freshly squeezed orange juice, left in the refrigerator for a few days, will have lost a significant amount of its vitamin C content. It is hard to know how much vitamin C we are getting from our food. Stress and smoking – a habit associated with stress – may affect our body's need for this vitamin. What better source to derive it from, than natural, pure honey?

As a point of interest, I have also found honey to be very effective in the healing of ulcers and burns. Many hospitals today are reverting to the use of honey in these cases, as it is a natural antibiotic, and I have yet to find anyone who is allergic to it.

Black molasses

Molasses is made from raw, unsulphured cane sugar. It is a black, treacle-like substance, packed with nutrients, and may be taken at any time when most convenient. I usually recommended a dose of one teaspoonful to be taken three times daily. Molasses can be taken undiluted, but if so, should be followed immediately by a drink of warm water as it has a tendency to discolour the teeth. I found one teaspoon of molasses dissolved in four ounces of warm water to be right for me. Taken like this, it is easily assimilated, more digestible, and it will not stain the teeth. Those with delicate stomachs, who may find that a teaspoonful is too much at one time, may take it in smaller, more frequent doses. If preferred, molasses can be taken on toast – wholemeal of course! There is very little nutrition in white bread, as the husk and kernel of the wheat have been extracted, leaving it deficient in fibre, vitamins and minerals.

Molasses may also be taken on porridge, or mixed with marmalade. However it is taken, as a food packed with iron and minerals, molasses is a wonderful blood-cleanser for arthritics. Like honey, molasses is also a marvellous external and internal healer. As I have said, arthritics are prone to suffer from stomach ulcers, diverticulitis, and similar conditions, caused by the acids eating away at the stomach and colon walls. As a rule, after taking molasses for one week, my patients report that these ailments are giving them less trouble. For external growths, boils, sores and cuts, molasses mixed with a little water and applied as a poultice is a wonderful, natural ointment. Molasses is also a laxative. Most people can take two teaspoons per day without experiencing any undue relaxation of the bowels, but as each case differs, I usually leave it to the individual to regulate his own intake. Used as a laxative, however, I always advise the patient to start with one teaspoonful per day, increasing the dosage, as the body becomes accustomed to it.

Like honey, molasses is a rich source of iron and can alleviate that tired feeling from which so many suffer. It is also a rich source of B vitamins, and so feeds the nerves, relieving spells of deep depression, bouts of painful neuralgia, and debilitating attacks of colds and influenza. Molasses also contains copper and magnesium, and is extremely high in pantothenic acid and inositol. Crude, raw, sugar cane molasses contains about fifty per cent fruit sugar, and can be used as a substitute for sugar on cereals and puddings, stirred into milk, or eaten in place of jam or jelly.

Molasses also contains a large amount of phosphoric acid and potassium. A combined deficiency of these in the body causes a breakdown of the cells, especially those of the brain and nerves. Anxiety uses up potassium salts in the blood and tissues and can produce a relapse in the treatment of arthritis. Here again, the taking of sugar cane molasses can be of great benefit, as it is very rich in potassium salts.

As I have mentioned before, an excess of uric acid in the body may give rise to gastric ulcers. The majority of medical practitioners realize that ulcers do not occur unless there is a deficiency of certain mineral salts in the tissues. Molasses replaces those mineral salts in the blood and tissues, thereby promoting a healing of the ulcers, wherever they may be. Many patients suffer from external ulcers, due to an attempt by the body to rid itself of toxic acids. Little can be gained from merely treating the local condition – a 'whole person' regime must be adopted. Thorough 'dietary cleansing' will remove the uric acid from the body, although a localized poultice of molasses and water may also be applied to good effect.

Many forms of skin disease are connected with arthritis, for example, eczema, dermatitis, psoriasis. 'Suppressive' ointment, firm favourites with the doctors, do much more harm than they do good. When applied to skin rashes and ulcers, they suppress the infection, driving it further into the body only to set up a more serious complaint elsewhere. Treatment of the 'whole person', through internal cleansing with molasses, can be of great help in dealing with these conditions, and external poultices of molasses will speed up the healing process.

High blood pressure, angina, and weak hearts, are very often associated with arthritis. These diseases have been known to respond extremely well to the 'molasses treatment'. Constipation and colitis are yet other conditions often connected with arthritis, and in these instances patients are normally advised to adopt a high-fibre diet. However, this is only half the story. Very often, a loss of muscle tone occurs, due to a lack of essential mineral salts in the body. Molasses proves most valuable in these cases, as the salts it contains help to re-establish muscle tone.

One distinguished doctor I know was of the opinion that if the sodium salts – which we absorb from our food and from table salt – are not counteracted by potassium salts, there will be a great risk of growths or arthritis developing. If potassium salt is taken into the body daily, it will help in the elimination of sodium salts, and thus minimize the danger. A good, natural way of getting potassium salt into the body, is through the taking of crude, black molasses.

Bathing in Epsom salts

The skin provides an excellent medium for the elimination of acid, and the use of Epsom salts as a 'drawing agent' cannot be too highly recommended. Epsom salts may be obtained in seven-pound bags, from chemists and, quite often from garden centres. I believe that roses benefit from the valuable mineral salts it contains.

There is nothing more relaxing than an Epsom salts bath at the end of a long, painful day, and the following method is my particular favourite:

1 Dissolve one pound (or three teacups) of Epsom salts in a bath of water as hot as you can bear it. (It should be noted that patients suffering from angina, high blood pressure, or any heart condition, should not use very hot water.) Do not add soap or bath cubes, salts or oils, as the alkalinity of these products will fight the acidity of the Epsom salts, thereby minimizing its effects.

2 Keep the water hot, by adding more from time to time, and start to exercise your joints. Beginning with the toes move them backwards and forwards; rotate the ankles clockwise and anti-clockwise; bend the knees and relax and stretch them; bend the spine backwards and forwards; bend and move the neck; rotate the arms clockwise and anti-clockwise; then exercise the fingers by clenching and unclenching the hand and then stretching the fingers as wide apart as possible. When exercising the fingers, a gentle, forceful movement is beneficial, as this helps to force out those acid deposits that have accumulated on the bones and between the joints.

3 The heat of the water will open the pores of the skin, enabling the Epsom salts to 'draw out' acid poisons. After ten to fifteen minutes, get out of the bath, dry yourself quickly with a warm towel, and get straight into a warm bed. The object of this is to keep the pores

of the skin open all night, to encourage the elimination of acid through sweating. Patients may find that sleeping between blankets will help to absorb the sweat.

This bath is a wonderful relaxer and pain-reliever, and a good night's sleep will usually be achieved. On rising, take a quick shower to wash away the accumulated acids and you will emerge refreshed and ready to face another day. It should be noted that this bath can be slightly weakening, and the patient may feel lethargic the following day. If this occurs, an hour's rest at midday will prove beneficial. For working arthritics, two baths, taken at weekends, may be advisable, and I certainly recommend that no more than three Epsom salts baths be taken per week.

On no account should the body be exposed to cold or draughts after this bath. This could lead to tension in the nerves and muscles, thereby causing pain and making matters far worse than before. Similarly, no work should be undertaken after the bath. Keeping warm is most important, as it will prolong the period of 'elimination'. A methodical 'pinching' of the skin, from the feet upwards, will help to increase circulation and improve muscle tone. However, under no circumstances, should this bath lead to exhaustion.

Of course, many arthritics are unable to get into the bath, and I suggest that they bathe hands and feet, as follows:

1 Take an ordinary kitchen bowl, and fill it with water as hot as you can bear.
2 Add to this one cupful of Epsom salts, and soak hands for ten to fifteen minutes.
3 Using forceful but gentle exercise, you will find it amazing how quickly movement is regained in previously locked joints.
4 Dry the hands, and wrap in a warm towel for five minutes to allow the pores to close.

5 Repeat this process with the feet.

These hand and feet baths may be taken three times daily or more often if possible. In many cases, some power will be regained in the hands within six weeks of regular treatment, and patients will find that they have the confidence to get in and out of the bath, without fear of falling. I once had a patient whose hands and fingers had become deformed and locked. In the course of four months of treatment, all this had disappeared. This lady was delighted to tell me that she could now open a tin of dog food without any difficulty. She is just one of the many who are daily experiencing similar results.

Very often, arthritics experience inflammation, pain, and swelling in various joints. A cold, wet pack will relieve this in a manner little short of miraculous. This should be carried out as follows:

1 Wring out some linen, or similar material, in cold water.
2 Wrap this around the affected part and cover with a woollen scarf or some warm flannelling.

This application will increase circulation to the affected part and draw out the pain and swelling, without the need to resort to any harmful drug. These natural treatments are often scornfully described as 'old wives tales'. However, their obvious merits should not be ignored in favour of drugs, which will only do you more harm in the long run.

The self-healing power of the body is really wonderful and nature is the only true healer. No matter what methods of treatment are employed, the body must, and always will, depend on the 'setting free' of the healing powers and forces within it. The essence of much disease is the accumulation of waste uric acid in the system, due to wrong dietetic habits. Elimination of these wastes is what nature is striving for, and therefore the tremendous value of the foregoing 'detoxication' programme should be obvious. Remember, good health has to be earned and worked for, but you will find the results well worth achieving.

Avoiding stress

First and foremost, the main requirement for ridding the body of arthritis, is positive thinking. This attitude of mind towards the success of the treatment is of paramount importance. Every member of the family can encourage the arthritic sufferer to adopt this attitude, and indeed, the diet that I recommend could prove beneficial to the family as a whole.

The avoidance of stress is also important. Stress is a commonly used term that is rather more easily recognized than explained. Because stress is really a personal condition, it can mean a number of different things to different people. In general, a person can be described as suffering from stress, when the pressures of work, family problems, money worries and so on, get beyond his ability to cope and thus ruin his peace of mind. These conditions invariably lead to impatience, irritability, depression, loss of concentration and sleeplessness.

Stress can also affect a person in a physical manner. Anxiety, fear and worry increase the body's production of chemicals called stress hormones. These can cause feelings of panic or discomfort in a normally healthy person, but to the arthritic, the outcome of the production of these hormones is often more serious. Stress hormones can raise the blood pressure, which in turn may lead to other complications. Stress is nothing new – living has always involved stress – but in recent times problems such as mass unemployment and the nuclear threat, as well as the daily strains of modern living, have greatly increased its effects.

There is some evidence that those most likely to suffer from stress often display similar personality traits. These people are usually impatient, ambitious, competitive and, as such, under constant pressure. A sudden, severe shock – such as news of a death in the family – has been known to cause a relapse in arthritis. This happened recently to a thirty-year-old patient of mine. She was progressing beautifully, ridding herself of her arthritis day by day. Suddenly, her father died, and the severe shock put her right back to square one.

Very often, there is no way of knowing if someone is suffering from stress. However, there may be 'tell-tale' signs, for example, heavier smoking and drinking habits, sudden over-eating, or loss of appetite. Sleeplessness, unaccountable tiredness, short temper, and an unusual difficulty in making decisions, are also signs of stress. Life is complicated, especially for the arthritic, but we often make matters worse for ourselves. For example, we often put ourselves under tremendous pressure by leaving things to the last possible minute. To avoid this, do everything you can at a reasonable pace, without hurrying. Plan ahead – give yourself plenty of time to shower and dress in the morning, and above all, do try to have a pleasurable, unhurried breakfast. This will ensure a good start to the day and set the pace for the following working hours. It is well worth getting up an hour earlier, in order to achieve this. To help avoid stress:

1 Take plenty of regular exercise, if possible – it is one of the best forms of relaxation.
2 Eat slowly, taking your mind off your work while doing so.
3 Find ways to 'escape' in your spare time, through books, pastimes, hobbies and sport.
4 Make sure you take a regular holiday. Do not make the excuse that you have not got time – make time!
5 Make sure you have enough rest – relaxation is vital. Some light reading at bedtime can help you to 'let go' mentally and physically before you go to sleep.
6 Try to avoid getting over-impatient; few things are

that urgent. If you really must get angry about something, try to get it out of your system by expressing your anger as quickly and honestly as possible.

7 Do not bottle up your anger, but try to find ways of getting rid of it.

8 Make sure that the goals you are trying so hard to achieve are what you really want. Ask yourself whether you need to be so competitive.

9 When you are anxious, make a special effort not to smoke or drink any more than usual. This will only be self-defeating in the long run, and the same applies to overeating.

10 Make a positive effort to change the things in your life that are a constant source of worry.

Having started the day supported by the power of positive thinking, you should now turn your thoughts to diet, and the eating of the correct foods necessary to the health of your body.

Rules for healthy eating

To the arthritic, an acid-free diet is of the utmost importance. However, the following dietary 'rules' are of value not only to the arthritic, but also prove beneficial to the overweight and those with heart conditions.

1 *Eat less salt*
Most of us eat much more salt than we need, and for some people, too much salt actually leads to increased blood pressure. Cut down on your salt intake, by:

- Using less salt in cooking.
- Never adding salt to prepared food.
- Choosing fresh, rather than processed foods.
- Avoiding salty foods, such as crisps, salted peanuts, etc.

2 *Cut out animal fats*
Butter, cheese, milk and cream are very high in lactic acid, and should be avoided altogether. They are also high in cholesterol and thus conducive to increased blood pressure. Cut down on your intake of fat, by:

● Using any vegetable margarine that is high in polyunsaturated fat.
● Using dried or skimmed milk.
● Eating cottage cheese – not to be confused with cream cheese, which is very high in lactic acid.

3 *Cut out all citrus fruits*
Oranges, lemons, grapefruit, and their juices, are full of citric acid. When combined with carbohydrates in the system, the result is a formation of uric acid. Pineapples, tomatoes, strawberries, plums, gooseberries and rhubarb are also high in acids, as are blackcurrants, red currants, blackberries and damsons. This also applies to fruit jams and marmalades, and to pickles made with malt or spiced vinegar. As a practical rule of thumb, if you think of a fruit and your mouth waters, it contains acid and should be avoided.

Unfortunately, citrus fruits provide a major source of vitamin C. This vitamin is of vital importance to the body and a lack of it can create iron deficiency, even leading to anaemia. It is essential, therefore, to take a good, naturally-produced vitamin C supplement each day, and I will enlarge on this at a later stage.

4 *Cut out 'old meats'*
Pork, beef, ham, bacon, sausages, pâtés, corned beef and similar prepared meats all contain old, fibrous tissue, full of acid. These days, when animals have a temperature, stomach upset, or minor ailment, they are pumped with antibiotics and other drugs, just as we are. When their meat is taken into our system, the residual 'poison' of those

drugs are also taken in, thereby setting up more problems for the already 'toxic' arthritic. Animals also eliminate acid waste from their bodies in much the same way as we do – through urination and bodily excretions. When they are killed for meat, this process of elimination stops suddenly. The acids seep back into the tissues, and when that meat is ingested, the animal's acids are ingested with it. The suffering arthritic has then got double trouble – not only his own toxic acids to get rid of, but also the acids of those animals as well. It therefore makes sense to avoid these meats whenever possible.

5 *Cut out alcohol*
All 'short' drinks are high in acid, and should be avoided. This applies to sherry, gin, whisky, vermouth, sparkling perry, all white and red wine – in fact, anything that has gone through a fermentation process.

6 *Cut out all fried foods, white sugar, and white bread*

7 *Avoid cream cakes and biscuits*

8 *Avoid all fruits bottled in syrup*

Foods for a healthy diet

There are a host of 'healthy' foods available to the arthritic, and it only takes a little thought and planning to ensure a well-balanced and varied diet. The following are some guidelines and suggestions for healthy eating:

1 Always buy 100 per cent wholemeal bread – you will find it more satisfying than white bread, and it is far better for you.
2 Choose a polyunsaturated, vegetable margarine.
3 Eat no more than three or four eggs per week.
4 Eat fresh, white fish – grilled, poached, baked, or

steamed, but never fried! Tinned fish, because of its invariably high salt content, is best avoided.

5 Eat plenty of cottage cheese, varying it with the addition of chives, spring onions, or chopped Spanish onions. Onions are a wonderful blood cleanser and a natural antibiotic. One tablespoon of raisins added to cottage cheese is another variation; also, fresh fruit, excluding of course, the ones that contain acid.

At lunch-time after a particularly busy morning in the clinic, I find that an easy, satisfying, tasty and nourishing meal can be made by adding sliced banana, apple, peach and a few raisins to a tub of natural cottage cheese.

6 Lamb may be eaten in moderation, and of course, the mint sauce can be made with cider vinegar – it tastes delicious! To sweeten the sauce, add one teaspoon of brown sugar or honey.

7 Eat chicken, duck, turkey, or indeed any fowl – although duck, being fatty, is less desirable.

8 Eat rabbit, lamb's liver, and heart. Kidneys, being an eliminative organ, should be avoided.

9 Eat plenty of fresh vegetables, raw or cooked. Salads are most beneficial, but do not add tomatoes, as they have a high acid content.

10 Choose fruits from among the many types that do not contain citric acid. For example, peaches, pears, bananas, apples, apricots, and melons.

11 Drinks, I am afraid, are limited. Apple juice, or any vegetable extract – for example, carrot juice – can be taken in unlimited amounts, but alcohol should be avoided, if possible. This is a bone of contention with many of my male patients. They ask, 'What can I have when I want a drink with my friends?' I usually recommend brandy with peppermint, or Guinness, as being the least harmful – but only in moderation! If one must have alcohol, it is advisable to take an extra

dose of cider vinegar, with or without honey, in order to cope with the extra acid intake. Many of my patients who are regular social drinkers ask the barman to make apple juice available to them, as they know they can drink this without any limitation. Of course, it is not intoxicating either, so they can drive home afterwards, without risk. No problems – and a double benefit!

12 Eat plenty of wholemeal cereals, and make your own pastries and cakes with wholemeal flour and low-fat margarine.

13 When buying food read the labels. Be very aware of what the product contains, and if there is anything in it that you should not have – put it back.

14 Cut down your intake of tea – it is full of tannic acid. If you must drink tea, make it weak. Also, use decaffeinated coffee, as ordinary coffee has a very high caffeine content.

You will find that the feeling of well-being, and the lessening of pain achieved by following these 'dietary rules', will have been well worth any sacrifice and effort involved.

Nutrition

I have found from my clinic that the vast majority of arthritics are extremely undernourished. Most are anaemic and suffer from stress and its related effects. I find that a good short cut to making them feel better is the administration of a first-class, natural source of vitamins and minerals, as follows:

1 I supply a good multivitamin and mineral tablet. This introduces a complete range of vitamins and minerals to nutritionally starved bodies. Coupled with instant protein powder, this is an excellent basis for a return to good health.

2 If patients are anaemic, I give additional iron.
3 If patients suffer from cramps and tingling sensations, I give calcium in tablet form.
4 I always recommend a vitamin C supplement, as the greatest source of this vitamin – citrus fruits – is not allowed.
5 Vitamin B complex is a must, as it feeds and soothes tired nerves, thus promoting a good night's sleep. Many people who come to the clinic already take one or other of the B vitamins, as they have been told that it is good for them. However, they do not realize that the taking of only *one* B vitamin, will create a deficiency of the other B vitamins in the body and can, therefore, cause more harm than good.
6 I find alfalfa extremely useful, and often give it to people who cannot take black molasses. Alfalfa seems to have similar properties and in my experience, very good results have been achieved through its use.

As I have stressed, over and over again, arthritis is a disease of dietetic origin, and as such, should be treated accordingly. The following chapter is designed to give the reader a further awareness of the importance of a good, wholesome diet.

4

Vitamins and Minerals – Their Uses in the Body

The more you study your nutrition, the more you learn about food, and the more you understand how your body works. Eating a lot does not necessarily mean getting the correct nourishment. More important than quantity is a variety of foods, that contain the correct amounts of proteins, minerals and vitamins needed to supply our bodies with enough energy for growth, repair and maintenance. The consequences may be serious if these vital nutrients are lacking.

Bulk and roughage are very important factors in the foods we eat, because without them the body cannot function properly and a state of acidosis may be set up in our bodies, leading to various chronic ailments.

The adoption of a plan of wholefood nutrition is essential to the good health and efficiency of the human body. When a wound is stitched or a broken bone is manipulated together, we all know that it is the body's own natural healing powers that heal the wound and mend the broken bone. We can also observe these natural healing powers at work in the case of colds or influenza, and in cases of fevers and inflammation. Usually in children and young people this is a very quick process, because at this stage in life the body's resistance is high and depletion of natural powers has not taken place. In older people, the healing is usually slower because the body's natural impetus towards health has been minimized, due to years of bad diet and abuse of the body through smoking, excessive alcohol and other pollutants. It is my belief that if all these instances were treated by the whole person elimination treatment which I advocate, not only would there be a swift return to normal health, but the patient would actually feel much better after than he did before the disease or wound occurred. This is because the body would have thrown off those harmful toxic acids and a clean, healthy body would have emerged.

Unfortunately, the long-suffering doctor, when called to the patient's bedside, is expected to perform a miracle and has no alternative but to give the patient a drug or antibiotic selected from the vast array available. The doctor has no time to explain to his patients that self-healing processes will go to work. The patient, however, may think that the GP just can't be bothered if he advises leaving the condition alone; but a programme of intelligent 'leaving alone' may be much better than medical intervention, which could be harmful. For years I have practised in my family a drugless campaign of treatment and this form of the promotion of my children's health has paid dividends. I maintain that a good diet supported by nutritional supplements in the form of protein, vitamins and minerals helps to promote good health and vigour.

Vitamins

'Vitamin' is a term applied to a group of substances which exist in minute quantities in natural food and which are necessary to normal nutrition, especially in connection with growth and development. Vitamin deficiency in the diet of young children and animals causes defective growth. In adults various diseases can arise, and persistent deprivation of one or other vitamin is apt to lead to a lower state of general health. Certain deficiencies in diet have been known to cause scurvy, beriberi and rickets.

Vitamin A
This vitamin is usually taken in more than ample quantity in a normal diet and is stored in the liver. It is developed originally by plants as a yellow colouring matter – carotene, for example, in carrots. It is also found in egg

yolk, liver, milk, butter and most green vegetables. The two richest sources of this vitamin are halibut liver oil and cod liver oil. The daily adult requirement of vitamin A is in the region of 4000 international units, though children and pregnant women have a higher requirement. Deficiency of vitamin A can be responsible for serious inflammation of the eyes known as 'xerophthalmia'; also for night blindness, various skin eruptions, defective development of the teeth and for want of vitality in the tissues, which could lead to localized inflammation. It is not destroyed by ordinary cooking processes.

Vitamin B_1

This is found in the husks of cereals and grains. Its deficiency may be produced by too careful milling of rice or by a diet of white bread to the exclusion of brown bread and other cereal sources of this vitamin. The resulting disease is a form of neuritis, with muscular weakness and heart failure. The best sources of this vitamin are wholemeal flour, bacon, liver, egg yolk, yeast and pulses. Pregnant women require more than the usual 0.5mg – a daily dose of 2mg is advisable.

Vitamin B_2

This is present in milk and is not destroyed during pasteurization. Other rich sources are eggs, liver, yeast and the green leaves of broccoli and spinach. It is also present in beer. Deficiency of this vitamin in the diet is thought to cause inflammation of the cornea, sores on the lips, and dermatitis. The minimal daily requirement for an adult is approximately 3mg but more is required during pregnancy and lactation.

Vitamin B_3

Little is known about this vitamin except that it is distributed widely in foodstuffs, both animal and vegetables. Yeast, liver and egg yolk are particularly rich sources. In rats, lack of this vitamin produces greying of the hair, but there is no evidence to show that this occurs in man. In chickens, lack of it causes dermatitis and degeneration of nerve fibres in the spinal cord.

Vitamin B6

This vitamin plays an important part in the metabolism of a number of amino acids. Deficiency leads to atrophy of the epidermis, the hair follicles and the sebaceous glands; neuritis may also occur. Young infants are more susceptible to deficiency than adults. They may lose weight, develop anaemia, and become very irritable; convulsions may also occur. Liver, yeast and cereals are rich sources of vitamin B6; fish is a moderately rich source, but milk and vegetables contain little. The minimum daily requirement in the diet is approx. 2mg.

Vitamin B12

This vitamin contains cyanide and cobalt. It was first isolated in 1948 and was found to be effective in the treatment of pernicious anaemia.

Brewers yeast is one of the richest sources of the B vitamins. Even so, it can take as much as 1kg. of yeast to yield some of the smaller dosages of B vitamins per capsule, currently quoted on the labels of natural vitamin supplements. Most of the B vitamins currently on the market are based on laboratory-synthesized chemicals, whether or not they are labelled 'natural'.

Vitamin C

This is especially found in fresh citrus fruits such as oranges, lemons, and grapefruits; also in green vegetables and, to a smaller extent, in milk, meat and other fresh foods. Canned vegetables, such as tomatoes, retain it as their reaction is acid. It is quickly destroyed by high temperature or by excess baking soda and other alkalis, and is gradually lost by oxidation in storage. Its deficiency leads to symptoms of scurvy, including muscular weakness, haemorrhages under the skin, swelling and inflammation of the gums, with loss of teeth, and serious damage to joints by haemorrhage. It can occur in babies fed persistently on artificial foods. The daily requirement of vitamin C is 30mg for adults and 60mg for children. It has been proposed that it is of value in the treatment of cancer, but there is no convincing evidence of its effectiveness.

Vitamin D

This vitamin is of special value for the growth of children, and its deficiency produces rickets, with softening and irregular growth of bones, so that swollen joints, distorted limbs, deformities of the chest, and similar malformations arise. Osteomalacia – a similar disease affecting the bones of adult women, results from the same causes when lime salts are absorbed from the bones during pregnancy. Rickets is also common among young dogs and other animals. It has long been known that cod liver oil was the chief remedy for rickets, and for a time it was supposed that its anti-rachitic action depended on vitamin A, but it is now known to be vitamin D. Only a few foods contain vitamin D naturally; they include cod liver oil and other fish oils. Egg yolk contains a smaller quantity; fats and milk contain very small quantities. Vitamin D aids in the absorption of phosphorus and calcium from the food, and increases absorption of these substances into the blood and bones. Bad effects may follow overdosage, because if too much calcium and phosphorus are maintained in the blood, the bones and teeth may become over-calcified and unduly hardened and calculi may form in the kidneys and other organs. The daily requirement for infants and nursing mothers is 400 – 800 international units, whilst for adults it is probably about 400 units.

Vitamin E

This is derived especially from the oil contained in seeds

and in green leaves, and small amounts are also present in other fresh foods. It is readily stored in the body and is unlikely to be found wanting in human beings, except in cases of very severe undernourishment and in premature babies. It is possible, however, that miscarriages may occasionally be due to its deficiency – in 1923 it was shown that a lack of this vitamin in rats caused failure to produce young. It is invaluable in the treatment of heart and blood disorders and it controls the unnecessary absorption of some nutrients. Our most reliable dietary sources are wholegrains, butter and margarine.

Vitamin K
This is the anti-haemorrhage vitamin, essential for the proper clotting of blood. It has been given successfully in cases of bleeding in infants and in cases of jaundice where there is a special tendency to bleeding. Bleeding in these conditions is thought to be directly due to deficiency in vitamin K. It is widespread in nature, the main sources being spinach, leafy vegetables, tomatoes and liver. The daily requirement has not been identified. Vitamin K deficiency occurs only in clinical situations, such as gall bladder, liver and intestinal disease. Deficiencies are not likely to occur today, since the vitamin is fairly well distributed in foods and the intestinal micro-organisms synthesize a considerable amount of it.

Iron
This is a metal which is an essential constituent of the red blood corpuscles, where it is present in the form of haemoglobin. It is also present in muscle and in certain respiratory pigments, which are essential to the life of many tissues in the body. Iron is absorbed principally in the upper part of the small intestine. It is then stored mainly in the liver and, to a lesser extent, in the spleen and kidneys, where it is available when required for use in the bone marrow, to form the haemoglobin in the red blood

corpuscles. The daily iron requirement is increased during pregnancy. Iron salts also have an astringent action, especially the chloride, and sometimes this property is made use of when it is used as a styptic to check bleeding.

Calcium

This is a metallic element present in chalk and other forms of lime. Although still commonly used in the treatment of chilblains, there is little evidence that calcium is of any real value in these conditions. It is a most important element in diet and the chief sources are milk and cheese. Calcium is especially needed by the growing child and the pregnant and nursing mother. The recommended daily intakes of calcium are 500 mg for children, 700 mgs for adolescents, 500–900 mg for adults and 1,200 mg for pregnant and nursing mothers.

Situations where calcium supplementation may be useful

1 Cataracts due to hypocalcaemia.
2 Allergies and elimination diets.
3 After the menopause, when oestrogen is lacking.
4 Toxic metal exposure (lead and aluminium).
5 Depression, anxiety, panic attacks, insomnia.
6 Muscle tics, twitches and cramps.
7 Joint and muscle aches, and arthritis.
8 Pregnancy and lactation.
9 Gastro-intestinal malabsorption.

Magnesium

This is one of the essential mineral elements in the body, without which it cannot function properly. The adult body contains around 25g, the greater part of which is in the bones. More than two-thirds of our daily supply comes from cereals and vegetables. As most other foods also contain useful amounts, there is seldom any difficulty in maintaining an adequate amount in the body. Deficiency leads to muscular weakness and interferes with the efficient working of the heart. Magnesium sulphate, commonly known as Epsom salts, is a saline purge. Epsom salts baths are used very effectively in the elimination of acids from the body, especially in cases of arthritis and rheumatism, and in fact any chronic disease, such as bronchitis or non-allergic asthma.

Choosing the right foods

Some people acquire dietary habits peculiar to their own fads and fancies, generally relying upon a large amount of filling foods, in complete ignorance of the known principles of nutrition. These habits may have a hereditary influence, because if a mother has not been sufficiently educated in the science of nutrition, to supply her family with healthy food, then there is very little hope that her daughter or son will be taught correct feeding habits, and so the story repeats itself.

In years gone by the bone-deforming disease of rickets was widespread in children throughout their formative years. Their diets were sadly lacking in the fruits and vegetables that provide vitamins and essential mineral salts, and in the absence of these foods, fevers raged and child mortality was high. Large quantities of nutritionally deficient foods are eaten today. The supermarket shelves are full of them and resistance to a change of diet is very persistent. Most of the deficiency foods are fattening and they tend to induce overeating. The refined carbohydrates are of this type – white flour, in its many forms of bread, cakes, pastries, biscuits, and pastas, and polished white rice. The introduction of the modern milling process means that the bran and germ of the wheat are rejected; the nutritionally rich parts of the wholegrain are excluded from the flour, and are sold separately as animal food or breakfast cereal. In this process there is a loss of valuable vitamins and minerals, especially those of the B complex, and also a loss of protein. Natural iron and calcium are among the minerals that are lost but now, by order of the government, iron is added to white flour in another form, as well as chalk to replace the absent calcium. It is stated that as many as twenty chemicals may be used in the production of the modern loaf of white bread. Such chemicals include bleaching agents to whiten the flour, preservatives, texturizers, anti-infection agents, emulsifiers and moisturizing agents. The white loaf is no longer the 'staff of life'. By far the best flour and bread to buy is 100 per cent wholemeal.

The well-being of the consumer depends entirely on the consumption of food in its pure natural state. In the case of flour, as with all other foods, it is a complex combination of substances that, when tampered with and some of the vitamins removed, is likely to be rendered completely valueless in terms of nutrition.

There is a direct relation between the consumption of wholefoods and the control of rheumatism and arthritis, and the springing up of wholefood shops around the country is not surprising. The problem remains that, although there is a crying need for wholefood nutrition, the public at large are ignorant of their requirements and do not know what to buy for their various illnesses. They buy vitamin E or whatever, because a friend told them it is good. Good for what they don't know and have no idea of where to find out. A resident dietician or nurse well versed in the uses of vitamins and minerals would be a tremendous boon, both to the health food store and the customer. People want to be healthy, but they don't know how to go about achieving that happy state; and directives from doctors, as a rule, are on the avoidance of specific foods.

White sugar is another threat to good nutrition. By the year 1700 the commercial refining of sugar had made it readily available and the consumption was 14lb per person per year. By 1800 the figure had risen to 16lb per person per year, and at present it runs at about 130lb per person per year. This commodity cannot be classed as food because it is completely devoid of all vitamins and minerals. One can become addicted to it; its chemical formula is not unlike that of alcohol. Sugar is a refined carbohydrate and dentists everywhere tell us that it is the principal cause of dental caries. It can be responsible for a vast array of other diseases, including obesity, diabetes, diseases of the intestine such as those very often found in conjunction with arthritis – colitis and diverticulitis; also constipation, haemorrhoids and varicose veins. All of these are blood disorders and directly related to rheumatism and arthritis.

Honey is often preferred to sugar because it is a more natural product than refined sugar. It has fewer calories, too – about 82 per ounce, compared with 112 for sugar. Analysis also shows that honey contains traces of many minerals and trace elements and some samples of honey also contain vitamins. To produce honey, the bee has partly digested complex sugars into simpler glucose and fructose sugars that are less disruptive to human blood sugar levels. Because honey is a natural product many health food shops carry a large selection. Taste is often the deciding factor in purchasing a particular type of honey. For those who like a light-coloured honey with a delicate flavour, acacia is a good choice. Set honey is traditionally used with teatime bread and butter, or breakfast toast. Liquid honey is easier for cooking or for use in drinks, remedies or natural beauty recipes. If you use honey for cooking it is best to choose one with a subtle flavour that will not overpower the other ingredients, and remember that honey is 20 per cent water.

Blended honey is the cheapest, because it is usually the product of more than one country. The most expensive honeys are single source honeys. These are produced by bees that have collected nectar wholly or mainly from one type of flower. The nectars give the honeys very distinctive flavours and colours.

'Pure' honey on a label means that the jar contains 100

per cent honey, even though it is blended, as opposed to a 'honey spread' product that contains sugar, syrups and other additives. Honey is the natural replacement for sugar – and much more beneficial to health.

Constructing a well-balanced diet

Disease is exactly what it says – DIS-EASE, and this means that for one reason or another the body is not *at ease*. If I cut my finger my whole body is in sympathy with that finger. Depending on the severity of the cut, there is a sudden shock, which will probably affect my nerves, giving me sleepless nights, which in turn will render me devoid of all energy and as a result my work will suffer. The reader will deduce from this statement that one simple action can bring about a chain of events, each one more serious than the other. In like manner, if we give a sweet, cake or pastry as a reward to a child for a job well done, or to stop him crying, it can trigger off a chain of events that may take years to come to fruition.

Similar symptoms may be related to a variety of conditions, most or all directly related to degenerative conditions in the body due to years of faulty dieting. Orthodox medical methods of treatment in the cure of arthritis and rheumatism have been unsuccessful because these diseases are systemic, due to years of bad diet, and nobody will succeed in the treatment of these diseases without an all-round promotion of health. There is no standard diet suitable for all individuals and identifying what is and what is not needed in any particular diet and supplemental nutrient pattern requires more than guesswork; although there is always an element of trial and error initially. Skilled observation, backed by extensive knowledge, chance observations using clues from questions and from the nutrient content of existing diets, experimentation with dietary improvement and nutritional supplements are all ways of determining a patient's nutritional deficiency. To rely on dietary adjustments alone when dealing with specific and unique needs of sick individuals and to ignore the proven need for supplementation, is a very futile exercise. I believe very strongly in supplementation, and I also believe in explaining in detail to my patients what various vitamin supplements will achieve for them. In alternative medicine as in life, it is by our fruits that we shall be known and judged.

Healing is really a very simple affair calling for love, discernment, wisdom and truth. The more complicated treatments are, the harder they are to understand and stick to. Hippocrates said that foods should be medicines and medicines food, and the true practitioner will discuss with his patient what foods, for whatever reasons, are poisonous to him. The practitioner may see the supplement as a nutrient but not so the patient who, in my experience, often sees it as a prop or substitute for balanced nutrition.

It should be clear from all this that there is nothing to equal a well-balanced diet. Experts say we must reduce intakes of fat, sugar and ordinary salt, and take more bread, potatoes, fresh vegetables and fruit. This is true no doubt, but you might add the considerations of quality and selection. *What kind of bread*? one may ask; we have to be careful with brown bread – it may have additives. *How were the vegetables grown*? Have they been sprayed or chemical fertilizers added? If so they may be completely devoid of the vitamins and minerals that are attributed to them. We should look to the fruit we eat: some people never eat fruit and this applies especially to arthritics, who cannot take citrus fruits. Here again it seems evident that some food supplements are necessary to our modern society. According to a report commissioned by the British Government, from a group of doctors and scientists, we need more wholefoods, real bread, fresh vegetables and fruit. What these present-day scientists are saying, in effect, is 'we are what we eat'. It seems to me that a gradual change is taking place in public thinking today, and despite the brainwashing of television and other advertising campaigns, the public are beginning to question the value of the average British diet, becoming more selective in their purchase of food and more aware of the ingredients it contains.

It takes a long time to adapt the body to any new or altered system of diet. If you are new to wholefoods, you should change to any new diet gradually. It is not necessarily wise to change your habits abruptly. The sensible plan is to move slowly and adapt to a natural diet by eating more and more foods that are not much altered from their natural state.

Meat
Meat is one of the foods most altered from its natural state by today's methods of factory farming. If you eat meat, quality – how the animals were reared, fed and slaughtered – must be of prime consideration.

Chicken One ounce of roast lean chicken gives 6.2g protein, 1.4g fat, 54 calories and no carbohydrate. Chicken is high in protein, low in fat and a very good source of iron and nicotinic acid. Vitamins B_1 and B_2 are also present.

The nutritional value of turkey is similar to that of chicken. Guinea fowl is also low in fat, while duck and goose are distinctly fatty. To lessen the fat content, remove the skin before eating roast meat.

Lamb The leanest lamb has only about 8 per cent fat. An ounce of lean roast lamb has only about 55 calories. Lean lamb is a very good source of iron.

Veal Veal is extremely lean, and is a very good buy for arthritics and the health conscious. A 3oz portion of veal has only 100 calories, but when roasted or fried, it has about 160. Lean veal has the same amount of protein and B vitamins as lean beef, but only half the iron.

There is nothing to equal a well-balanced diet to ensure bodily health and mental vigour, and in searching for a healthy way of eating, many people decide to cut down on the amount of meat they eat and find some other sources of protein.

Fish
Fish has a lot to offer. It may still be an animal food, but the fat it contains is polyunsaturated, unlike that of other animal products. Polyunsaturated fatty acids have been shown to have a beneficial effect on the fats in the bloodstream. Their presence helps to reduce the deposit of saturated fats causing narrowing and hardening of the arteries and contributing to heart disease. Fish, in particular oily fish, like mackerel and herring, offer special types of marine oils that make the blood less likely to form clots which cause thrombosis in the narrowed arteries. Both oily fishes and white fish contain valuable vitamins A and D. White fish need extra oil or liquid added during cooking, but oily fishes do not because their oil content enables them to 'cook themselves'. Wrapped in spinach to keep the steam in and prevent them from drying, they make an excellent and very easy meal. Recent research has shown that the dramatic drop in the amount of fish eaten in Britain can be correlated to the rise in heart disease. Populations like the Eskimos who eat large amounts of seal meat are free from heart disease.

Although fish provides protein, it does not provide fibre, and as a lack of this prevents the bowel functioning properly, some form of fibre should be added to the meal – for example, vegetables or fruit, or both.

Porridge
This is apparently the new wonder food. At least, that is what American doctors are now saying. They have found that it helps to regulate both blood sugar levels and fats. So in the USA porridge is now being recommended for the

treatment of diabetes, and in some cases for prevention of diabetes, high blood pressure and heart disease. Oats contain a gummy substance – beta glucens – which is very evident when you are boiling them up yourself. This can apparently reduce blood cholesterol levels by a third, as well as reducing blood sugar and fats. Oat bran is particularly rich in this fibre-based material and porridge oats, being the whole rolled oats, contain all of its natural fibre. Doctor James King, of the University of Kentucky says of the work being done on oats and porridge: 'This is the first time that anyone has demonstrated that a particular food can lower blood cholesterol. It is not uncommon for someone to come into our hospital with a blood cholesterol count of 300, and go out with a level of 195, which is relatively safe'. When the gummy fibre from oats reaches the colon, it is fermented by bacteria which produce fatty acids. These acids are absorbed into the bloodstream and have the effect of shutting down the body's production of sugar (glucose), which is made from starch and fats. This action lowers and stabilizes the level of blood sugar, a result which is, of course, especially beneficial to diabetics. In any case, oats have traditionally been known as a food for stamina and strength. This new work underlines the value of this important cereal in any really healthy diet. From now on we should look at porridge with the reverence that our forefathers did, and perhaps we would be much healthier for doing so.

Fibre

Bran is the richest source of all dietary fibres. A fibre rich diet, including bran, is highly desirable, and acts as a preventive measure against diverticulitis. This is a disease of the colon and constipation is now recognized as its underlying cause; bran is very often used in the treatment of diverticulitis. Any dietary substance which retards the absorption of carbohydrates may be beneficial to the body, and in this respect dietary fibre is seen to be a very valuable commodity. A large proportion of people develop difficulty in utilizing carbohydrates in their diets during middle age. This difficulty is caused by a fault in the insulin production of the body. Insulin is known to control excess blood sugar and if this rises too high, sugar appears in the urine and the person is diagnosed as diabetic. A group very closely related to diabetics is the group classified as having 'impaired glucose tolerance'. Lack of dietary fibre may also be the cause of varicose veins, due to abdominal pressure caused by straining when constipated, and also haemorrhoids, for the same reason. Dietary fibre plays a very beneficial role in the stabilizing or correction of these ailments.

A fibre-rich diet for children encourages mastication of food and helps to keep the teeth clean. The old saying 'an apple a day keeps the doctor away' is proved today to be a very wise saying; it does keep the doctor away, and the dentist too. An apple is a wonderful source of fibre. An adequate intake of all nutrients is essential for health and activity, and there are additional requirements for growth, pregnancy, lactation and in times of stress, such as infection. The exact amounts needed are different for each individual, and depend not only on such readily quantifiable factors as height, weight and sex, but also on physical activity throughout the day, the rate of internal activities, such as heart beat and the climate.

I hope that the reader will now be convinced that a good, healthy diet is the essence of physical well-being, and realizes that without it, the body will go into a state of dis-ease. 'Prevention is better than cure' the saying goes – how true. Once the body reaches that sad state of disease, a very determined effort is needed to help it to regain that happy state of profound health that is its birthright. To sum up, I remind you that a daily diet for healthy living should contain the following:

Protein The material of life, found in meats, poultry, fish and dairy products.

Fats In the form of polyunsaturated oils – corn oil, peanut oil etc. Plants are the best wholefood source of polyunsaturated fats.

Carbohydrates To supply us with heat and energy; taken in the form of bread, potatoes, rice and pastas.

Vitamins, minerals and trace elements From a variety of sources, as expained earlier in this chapter.

Roughage or fibre From apples, green vegetables, bran and oats.

The whole person elimination treatment, which I referred to early on, I have practised in my family for years. When any of the family developed influenza or bronchitis, I treated them as follows, with excellent results:

Two days on orange juice only.
Two days on fresh fruit only.
On the 5th day, fresh fruit plus half a glass of milk for breakfast, lunch and dinner.
On the 6th day a little wholemeal bread was introduced and green salad; and from then on a gradual resumption of normal diet.

In the case of lung congestion an Epsom salts bath is invaluable. This bath draws the congestion away from the lungs and, as I said before, it is an excellent medium for eliminating uric acids by drawing them out through the skin. The patient gets instant relief.

5

Recipes for Arthritis Sufferers

The power of positive thinking is invaluable in getting rid of any disease and arthritis is no exception. Always remember to direct your thoughts away from the fact that you have got arthritis, and instead direct them towards achieving good health. Every morning when you wake up think, 'This is another day, when I have another opportunity to make myself feel better'. Picture yourself as radiantly healthy and then go all out to achieve it, especially through your diet.

Eating the acid-free way is healthy for the whole family and especially for those suffering from heart trouble, high blood pressure or angina, because an acid-free diet is very similar to a low-fat diet, except that citrus fruits and fruit juices are forbidden. However, there is a whole host of foods that you can have without feeling deprived. Healthy eating certainly need not be boring.

Remember to keep away from saturated fats. These are easy to recognize as they remain hard at room temperature – lard, suet, butter, dripping, white cooking fat, hard margarine and, of course, fat from meat.

The fat contained in cheese, cream and milk is exactly the same as the fat contained in butter – it is saturated. Cream cheeses and hard cheeses such as Stilton and Cheddar are very rich in fat, as are double cream and whipping cream. Shop-bought biscuits, pastries, cakes, puddings, sauces and soups invariably contain a very high content of fat. Some vegetable margarines are also highly saturated, so it is wise to read all labels and be aware of what any product contains before you buy it.

The following are ways of cutting down on saturated fat:

1 Cut out all dairy products – butter, cheese, milk and cream.
2 Always use skimmed milk or dried milk, in tea, coffee or any recipe demanding milk.
3 Always choose low-fat cheese – cottage cheese is very good because, although the fat has been taken away, it contains proteins, vitamins and minerals.
4 Before you cook meat, cut away all obvious fat.
5 Use sunflower margarine as a substitute for butter.
6 Make your own pastries, cakes and biscuits, using sunflower margarine where the recipe advises hard margarine or butter.
7 Use sunflower oil for basting roasts and grills, for browning meat and vegetables, and for mixing sauces and dressings.
8 Include some oily fish in your menus, but always remember to drain excess oil from canned fish such as tuna, sardines and salmon, herrings and mackerel, because it is added oil and not the polyunsaturated oil from the fish.
9 Go for plain or dry-roasted nuts if you can find them, but don't indulge in cashews, coconuts or salted crisps and peanuts.

Many arthritics suffer from heart trouble, high blood pressure, angina or gallstones, and these people would be well advised to keep to low-cholesterol foods. Cholesterol is a fat-like substance, not a true fat, and it is found in all foods of animal origin. Offal, kidney, liver and heart, and egg yolks are all very rich in cholesterol. Shellfish, especially prawns and shrimps, have a high cholesterol content, as does fish roe, and high fat dairy foods such as cream and butter.

Eggs are not a good alternative to meat and fish and three eggs a week are adequate for people with any form of blood disorder. Remember to count all the hidden eggs in the dishes you prepare – cakes, puddings and sauces, for example.

Casseroling is a good cooking method: the flavours of the ingredients have time to mellow and you can skim off every trace of fat once the casserole has gone cold. Use puréed root vegetables – carrots, parsnips, potatoes – as thickeners; they do much less damage than cream or egg yolks.

When eating out, keep your menu simple – fresh fruit is a good starter, or consommé. It is best to avoid creamy soups, pâtés, shellfish, or anything fried. Chicken, fish, or lamb are good for a main course. Always avoid fried foods or pastries – they will probably be prepared with a saturated fat. Finish your meal with sorbet or fruit. A little meringue without cream would be acceptable, or different kinds of fresh fruit, though not citrus fruits.

A fresh green salad every day is a must for the arthritic, plenty of lettuce, spring onions or spanish onions, radishes, green and red peppers, chicory, celery, grated carrot, grated cabbage, etc. Add some natural cottage cheese and you have a delightful, health-giving meal.

There is no need to make any radical changes in your eating habits – just eat wholesome foods that contain as much goodness as possible and the least amount of harmful acids, such as tannic acid from tea and coffee. Switch to herbal teas and decaffeinated coffee; if you must have tea or coffee, have it weak. It is most important also to avoid lactic acid, the main sources of which are butter, cheese, milk and cream. Also, of course, the citric acid contained in citrus fruits and juices and, in fact, any acid fruit. It pays to have the best; most people today are beginning to take a second look at the food they eat and are becoming very aware of what is printed on the label.

A good breakfast

As I carry out my daily work in the clinic I meet a lot of patients with digestive problems – hiatus hernia, stomach ulcers, diverticulitis. When I ask them to give me a run down on their daily diet, invariably I am told: 'I never have breakfast; perhaps I will have a cream cracker and a little cheese for lunch, but I always have a good large evening meal when the family come home.' The habit of eating one big meal a day, and especially in the evening, is all wrong. It is an excellent way of raising the blood pressure and putting up blood fats. A protein-rich breakfast will stop that sinking feeling by raising the blood sugar and keeping one alert, thereby giving a good energy output and a feeling of being able to cope with the day's stresses and strains. Wholegrain cereal with a little dried fruit, skimmed or powdered milk and the addition of bran is quite delicious and very satisfying. Later in this chapter I will give a selection of nourishing breakfasts. Eating is a very necessary part of living and it is most important that we enjoy what we eat. Getting up an hour earlier in the morning pays dividends. It takes the tension out of the beginning of the day and provides us with enough time to sit down and have a leisurely breakfast, masticating the food properly without having to keep an eye on the time. Of course, wholefood eating cuts out 'empty' calories (i.e. those that make fat) and provides the body with what it needs to burn up excess fat. Changes in diet need self discipline, but the rewards are many.

A lot of people drink cup after cup of tea in the morning, but as this stimulates the secretion of gastric juices it should be avoided by people suffering from stomach ulcers. The digestion of starch is delayed in the stomach by the taking of too much tea; also, of course, it is full of tannic acid and for arthritics in particular, this is most undesirable.

Coffee contains a drug called caffeine which in my opinion is an unnatural stimulus for the heart. It dilates the blood vessels in the skin so people suffering from inflamed skin conditions should avoid it altogether. Glaucoma sufferers should not take it because it affects the blood vessels in the eyes. Addiction to coffee is not unusual; I had a female patient in the clinic a short time ago who has nine strong cups of coffee a day – she looked horrified when I asked her to cut it down. She told me that she had run out of her favourite brand about a week previously and experienced tremors, high temperature, migraine, irritability and nervousness. She couldn't go to bed without borrowing some coffee from a friend – then she recovered and her symptoms vanished. Ground coffee contains about 150mg of caffeine; instant coffee contains about 90mg. I always advise my patients to switch to decaffeinated coffee which only contains about 3mg, and I also advise herbal teas, which are quite harmless and a very beneficial alternative.

In the following pages you will find a variety of breakfast dishes that can safely be adopted by the arthritic or the heart sufferer. I put porridge oats first as a breakfast – a natural food and still one of the cheapest, yet one of the most wholesome and well balanced foods available for children and adults alike. Porridge is easily prepared, involving very little effort and furnishing the arthritic with a good, warming start to the day.

In the following recipes, where milk is mentioned, use skimmed or reconstituted powdered milk. For margarine, always use sunflower or polyunsaturated vegetable margarine.

Basic breakfast
To make porridge, stir one cupful of porridge oats into a saucepan containing three cups of milk or water. Add 1 teaspoon sea salt and bring to the boil, stirring continuously; then simmer for 4 minutes, stirring occasionally. The porridge is now ready to serve. One or two teaspoons of molasses sugar may be added if desired.

Egg yolks are a cholesterol-rich food so it is best to limit your egg intake to two or three per week, and adopt other ideas for breakfast. A glass of apple juice, or some stewed apple with a little muesli, is a good idea. Follow this with wholemeal bread rolls, toast or bran muffins spread with a polyunsaturated margarine or honey. A pleasant alternative for breakfast is a carton of low fat yoghurt and fresh fruit in season.

Breakfast Sunshine
  4 tablespoons rolled oats
  1 banana, sliced
  1 tablespoon honey
  1 teaspoon sunflower oil
  2 oz sultanas
  1 oz almonds, chopped
  skimmed milk

Method Mix all ingredients together and serve with skimmed milk. Serves two.

Bran Muffins
  4 oz wholemeal flour
  2 teaspoons baking powder
  ½ teaspoon sea salt
  3 oz bran
  1 tablespoon wheatgerm
  ½ oz soft brown sugar
  1 egg, size 4
  1½ pint skimmed milk
  4 tablespoons sunflower oil

Method Brush twelve deep bun tins with oil. Place dry ingredients in a bowl. Beat egg in a basin with milk and oil. Add to dry ingredients and mix together. Fill each bun tin with the mixture and bake in hot oven, 200°C (400°F) gas mark 6, for 25–30 minutes. Serve warm, spread with sunflower margarine and honey if desired.

Honey Muesli
  2 tablespoons rolled oats
  1 apple, grated
  1 tablespoon honey

½ cup natural yoghurt or skimmed milk
Chopped nuts

Method Mix all ingredients together, stirring well, and serve immediately. Makes two servings. Instead of oats other cereals may be used; cracked wheat, barley kernels or some wheatgerm may be added, sunflower seeds, raisins or slices of banana.

Oatmeal Breakfast Cakes
   2 oz rolled oats
   1 oz plain flour
   ¼ teaspoon bicarbonate of soda
   ½ pint skimmed milk
   1 egg
   1 teaspoon Australian clear honey
   Corn oil for frying

Method Mix together the dry ingredients. Beat egg with honey. Stir egg mixture into dry ingredients, then slowly add milk, stirring well. Heat a little oil in a frying pan and drop in tablespoons of the pancake batter, spaced well apart. Cook over a moderate heat. When the top is just set and underside golden, turn and cook the second side. Serve hot with sunflower margarine and honey. These pancakes make a pleasant change from the usual breakfast toast. Makes 18–20 pancakes.

Fruit Salad
   1 apple, chopped
   1 sliced banana
   A few grapes
   1 small tin of peaches or pears in their own juice (not in syrup)

Method Combine all ingredients and serve with a slice of wholemeal toast and sunflower margarine.

Baked Custard
   1½ cups skimmed milk
   1 tablespoon honey
   2 eggs
   Vanilla essence

Method Beat eggs and honey, add skimmed milk and vanilla essence. Pour into a pie dish lightly greased with margarine. Cook gently, standing in a dish of water, until set. Serve with a round of wholemeal toast.

Egg Rolls Toasted
   2 eggs
   ½ oz sunflower margarine
   1 tablespoon skimmed milk
   Worcester sauce
   Thin slices wholemeal bread, spread with margarine
   A little pepper and a pinch of sea salt

Method Melt the margarine in a small saucepan, blend in the beaten egg with the seasoning and sauce, stir well until scrambled. Remove the crusts from the wholemeal bread and spread the scrambled egg on to the plain side. Roll up and place under the grill, toasting evenly all round 3–5 minutes.

Eggs with Mushroom Stuffing
   ¾ cup chopped mushrooms
   2 teaspoons parsley
   4 hard-boiled eggs (halved)
   4 oz cottage cheese
   Worcester sauce
   Sunflower margarine

Method Fry the prepared chopped mushrooms with the parsley in a little margarine. Remove the yolks from the hard-boiled eggs and mash them with the mushroom mixture, adding Worcester sauce and seasoning to taste. Fill the halved egg whites with the stuffing and place in a greased fireproof dish. Cover with cottage cheese. Place under a pre-heated grill for 5–10 minutes.

Fluffy Egg Nests
    6 eggs
    6 slices hot wholemeal toast,
       spread with sunflower margarine
    Sea salt and pepper

Method First prepare the toast. Separate the eggs, leaving the yolks in the half-shells until required. Season the whites and beat them until stiff enough to form peaks. Pile the egg whites round the outer edges of the toast slices and drop the yolks into the centre. Season again. Place under a pre-heated grill and cook gently until the yolks are firm and the whites delicately tinged with brown. Serve on a hot dish and garnish with parsley. Serves six.

Grilled mushrooms
    Fresh mushrooms
    Slices of wholemeal toast, spread with sunflower mar-
       garine
    Pepper and a little sea salt
    Nutmeg

Method Wash the mushrooms, removing the skin and stalks. Brush with margarine and sprinkle with sea salt, pepper and a little nutmeg. Place under a pre-heated grill, cap side up. Cook for 8–10 minutes. Serve on wholemeal toast.

Turkey Sausage Rolls
    8 turkey sausages
    Sunflower margarine
    8 slices wholemeal bread, thinly cut

Method Grill the sausages. Remove the crusts from the bread, spread with margarine and roll a sausage in each slice of bread, margarine-side inwards. Place under the grill and toast evenly all round. This dish can be served with scrambled eggs or mushrooms.

Stuffed Turkey Sausages
    10 turkey sausages
    10 thin slices of lamb's liver
    Melted sunflower margarine
    2 cups wholemeal breadcrumbs
    1 small onion
    A pinch each of sea salt and pepper
    2 teaspoons sage

Method Mix together the crumbs, finely chopped onion, sage and seasoning and bind with melted margarine. Split the sausages lengthwise and spread with the stuffing. Wrap each in a very thin slice of lamb's liver and secure with a cocktail stick. Place under a pre-heated grill and cook for approximately 10 minutes, turning as required. Serve at once.

Honey Butter
    4 oz sunflower margarine
    4 level tablespoons honey

Method Cream the margarine and gradually add honey. Beat well together until light and fluffy. Keep in a sealed jar, for use on wholemeal bread, toast or biscuits. Chopped nuts or raisins can be added.

Honey and Ginger Spread
    4 oz honey butter (see previous recipe)
    2 level tablespoons chopped preserved ginger
    2 level tablespoons chopped toasted almonds

Method Add ginger and almonds to the honey butter and mix well. Serve with wholemeal bread or toast.

Grilled fish dishes

Carp
    2–3 lb carp
    ⅓ cup sunflower oil
    A pinch of sea salt
    Pepper
    Parsley for garnish

Method Prepare the fish by cleaning, scaling and washing. Split open and marinate in the oil for 15 minutes. Cook under pre-heated grill for about 20 minutes, turning once only. Season and serve garnished with parsley.

Cod with Olives
    1 lb fresh cod fillet
    1 oz sunflower margarine
    Toasted crumbs (wholemeal)
    1 egg
    Olives

Method Prepare the cod by cleaning and cutting into small portions; coat with egg and crumbs. Place in a fireproof dish and dot with margarine. Place under a pre-heated grill for 10 minutes. Garnish with olives and serve.

Cod with Mushrooms
    1 lb cod fillet
    2 oz mushrooms
    Sea salt and pepper
    ½ oz sunflower margarine
    ¼ lb creamed potatoes
    Parsley

For the sauce
¼ pint stock
½ oz sunflower margarine
½ oz wholemeal flour

Method Prepare the cod and cut into small pieces. Place in a greased fireproof dish and sprinkle with a little sea salt and pepper. Add some of the chopped mushrooms. Cover the fish with stock and dot the top with knobs of margarine. Bake in a moderate oven, 190°C (375°F)/gas mark 5, for about 30 minutes. Strain off the liquid and use it to make a basic sauce with the fat and flour. Season to taste. Piped creamed potatoes round the edge of the dish. Place under a hot grill for 10–15 minutes to brown the top. Serve garnished with parsley.

Grilled Haddock
1 medium-sized haddock
1 oz sunflower margarine
½ oz wholemeal flour
A little sea salt and pepper

Method Wash and trim the fish. Brush it over with melted margarine and turn it in the seasoned flour. Place under a pre-heated grill and cook gently for 15 minutes, turning once. Serve on a hot dish garnished with parsley.

Lobster with Toast
1 medium-sized lobster
¼ pint white sauce
2 rounds toast (dry)
Olive oil
3 oz cottage cheese

Method Prepare lobster by slitting down underside from head to tail. Remove the soft shell on the underside of the tail and flatten out the lobster as much as possible. Remove insides and discard them. Remove flesh from claws. Cut the flesh into pieces and mix it with 2 tablespoons white sauce, adding a little sea salt and pepper to taste. Wash shell thoroughly and rub with oil. Return the mixture to the shell and top it with cottage cheese. Grill until golden brown. Place filled shell in the centre of an oval dish and garnish with triangles of toast.

Grilled Salmon
    Fresh salmon slices
    Corn oil
    Spring onions, chopped
    Melted sunflower margarine
    Chopped parsley
    1 or 2 anchovy fillets

Method Marinate the seasoned slices of salmon for about one hour in a mixture of corn oil, spring onions and parsley. Drain them well and brush both sides with melted margarine. Grill for approximately 10 minutes. Turn the slices over and cook for a further 5 minutes. Place the anchovy fillets on them and continue cooking for about 5 minutes. Serve with creamed potatoes and peas.

Summer Fish Dish
    4 cod steaks
    1 tablespoon cider vinegar
    For the sauce
    6 oz diced mushrooms
    4 tablespoons natural yoghurt
    2 oz cottage cheese
    A little sea salt and pepper
    Cucumber slices and parsley for garnish

Method Place cod in an ovenproof dish and cover it with cider vinegar. Cook in the centre of a pre-heated oven, 180°C (350°F) gas mark 4, for 20–25 minutes. Mix all the sauce ingredients together and pour it over the cod steaks. Garnish with cucumber slices and parsley. Serve with new potatoes glazed with margarine and salad.

Plaice and Apple Bake
    4 fillets of plaice, skinned
    ½ oz sunflower margarine
    1 tablespoon cider vinegar
    Parsley for garnish
    For the filling
    1 small apple, peeled and sliced
    1 small green pepper, seeded and halved
    4 oz cottage cheese
    A little black pepper

Method Chop half the apple and half the pepper (slice the remainder of each for garnish). Combine together all the filling ingredients. Spread some on each of the fillets and roll them up. Place together in a casserole and dot with margarine. Pour on the cider vinegar and cover. Cook in the centre of pre-heated oven, 190°C (375°F) gas mark 5, for 40 minutes. Garnish with parsley and slices of pepper and apple. Serve with green beans and new potatoes glazed with melted margarine.

Stuffed Trout with Almonds
    4 medium-sized trout, cleaned and gutted
    For the stuffing
    3 oz sunflower margarine
    1 small onion peeled and finely chopped
    4 oz wholemeal breadcrumbs
    2 oz raisins
    1 dessertspoon cider vinegar
    2 sticks celery, chopped
    2 tablespoons finely-chopped parsley
    2 oz flaked almonds
    A little sea salt and freshly ground black pepper

Parsley for garnish

Method Wash the trout in cold water and wipe dry. Melt 1 oz margarine and sauté the onion until soft but not brown. Place the breadcrumbs, raisins, onion, cider vinegar, celery, parsley and ½ oz almonds in a bowl and mix together thoroughly. Season and then fill the trout with this stuffing. Place the trout on a foil-covered dish. Dot with the remaining margarine and sprinkle with flaked almonds. Cover with foil and bake in a pre-heated oven, 180°C (350°F) gas mark 4, for about 1 hour or, depending on the size of the trout, until the flesh is tender. Place on serving dish and garnish with parsley. Serve with boiled potatoes, glazed with margarine, and a green vegetable.

Fish and Pasta Salad
    12 oz smoked haddock, cooked, boned and flaked
    4 oz packet frozen french beans, cooked according to
      instructions
    6 oz pasta sheils, cooked in boiling salted water for 13
      minutes and drained
    4 oz mushrooms, washed and sliced
    2 tablespoons parsley
    For the dressing
    4 tablespoons sunflower oil
    2 tablespoons cider vinegar
    ¼ teaspoon dry mustard
    A pinch of demerara sugar
    A little sea salt and pepper

Method Place all dressing ingredients in a screw top jar and shake for a few seconds until thoroughly mixed. Mix together in a bowl all salad ingredients and toss in the dressing.

Mackerel Pizza
    For the scone base

1 oz sunflower margarine
2 oz wholemeal flour
2 oz plain flour, sieved
½ teaspoon baking powder
½ teaspoon sea salt
½ teaspoon mixed herbs
1 egg, size 4
1 tablespoon milk
For the topping
½ oz sunflower margarine
1 onion, peeled and chopped
3 oz mushrooms, trimmed and chopped
7½ oz can mackerel, drained and flaked
A pinch of oregano
3 oz cottage cheese
Green olives, sliced, for garnish

Method Place all ingredients for scone base in mixing bowl and use wooden spoon to mix. Turn on to lightly floured surface and knead gently. Shape into flat round, 8–9 in in diameter, and place on a baking sheet. Melt margarine and sauté onion and mushrooms. Add mackerel and oregano and spread over scone base. Spread cottage cheese on top and garnish with olives. Bake in hot oven, 200°C (400°F) gas mark 6, for 20–25 minutes. Serve hot or cold with a green salad.

Kipper Pâté
2 kippers
4 oz curd cheese
A pinch of cayenne pepper
A little sea salt and black pepper
1 tablespoon natural yoghurt

Method Poach kippers in water for 5–6 minutes and let them cool slightly in the liquid. Remove skin and bones. Place kipper flesh and remaining ingredients in a liquidizer and blend until smooth. Pile into a dish and serve with wholemeal toast spread with margarine.

Meat Dishes

When buying meat choose the leanest and before cooking it, trim off any visible fat; expensive cuts are not necessary. When browning meat and vegetables for casseroles, use sunflower oil.

Lamb Kebabs

12 oz leg lamb, trimmed and cut into 1½ in cubes
4 oz button mushrooms
1 green pepper, de-seeded and cut into 1 in squares
8 bay leaves (optional)
Sunflower oil

Method Arrange lamb cubes, mushrooms, peppers and bay leaves on four long skewers. Brush with oil and place under a pre-heated grill for 10–12 minutes, turning and brushing regularly. Serve with boiled rice and mixed salad.

Lamb and Potato Curry

2 oz clarified sunflower margarine
2 onions, finely chopped
1 clove garlic, crushed
1½ in piece fresh root ginger, peeled and chopped
1 teaspoon turmeric
1 tablespoon ground coriander
¼ teaspoon hot chilli powder
1 teaspoon ground cumin
1 tablespoon cardamon seeds, crushed
½ teaspoon ground cloves
2 lb lean lamb steaks, cubed
15 fl oz water
1 teaspoon sea salt

2 bay leaves
1 lb small potatoes, scrubbed

Method Melt the margarine in a large saucepan. Add the onions and garlic and fry until golden brown. Stir in the ginger and chilli powder and fry for 4 minutes, stirring frequently. Add a spoonful or two of water, if the mixture becomes dry. Add the meat cubes and fry until evenly browned. Stir in the water, salt and bay leaves and bring to the boil. When the mixture begins to bubble, reduce the heat to a low simmer for 1¼ hours. Add the potatoes and bring to the boil again. Cover and simmer for another 45 minutes, or until the meat is cooked through and tender. Transfer the mixture to a warmed serving dish and serve at once. Makes four to six servings.

Lamb Kebabs with an Indian Flavour
    1 medium-sized onion, peeled and chopped
    3 garlic cloves, crushed
    1½ in piece of fresh root ginger, finely chopped
    2 green chillis, finely chopped
    2 tablespoons chopped coriander leaves
    3 tablespoons natural yoghurt
    ½ teaspoon turmeric
    1 tablespoon cider vinegar
    1 teaspoon sea salt
    ½ oz fresh breadcrumbs
    1½ lb minced lamb
    1 oz melted sunflower margarine
    Cucumber slices for garnish

Method Combine all ingredients, except the cucumber, in a large bowl. Knead until the ingredients are blended and the mixture is stiff. Leave to stand for 30 minutes. Pre-heat the grill to high. Lightly grease twelve skewers with a little of the melted margarine. Dampen hands and remove small pieces of the meat mixture and shape them around the skewers. Put the skewers on a lined grill pan and brush with half the remaining margarine. Grill for 5 minutes. Turn over, brush with the remaining margarine and grill for another 5 minutes. Arrange the skewers on a bed of boiled rice and garnish with slices of cucumber. Serve at once.

Lamb Maryland
1½ cups skimmed or made-up dried milk
¼ cup seasoned flour
4 lean lamb chops
1 egg, lightly beaten with a teaspoon of water
1½ cups fresh breadcrumbs
8 tablespoons sunflower margarine
3 tablespoons sunflower oil
½ teaspoon honey
1 tablespoon wholemeal flour

Method Pour 4 tablespoons of milk into a saucer and put the seasoned flour into a shallow dish. Dip the lamb chops into the milk, then into flour, and shake off any excess. Set the chops aside for 10 minutes to allow the coating to dry slightly. Put the egg mixture into one dish and the breadcrumbs in another. Dip the chops one at a time into the egg and then in the breadcrumbs, shaking off any excess. Melt 6 tablespoons of margarine with the oil in a frying pan. Add the chops and cook over a low heat, turning occasionally, for 20 minutes or until they are cooked through. Transfer to kitchen towels to drain, cover and keep hot while you prepare the sauce. Melt the remaining margarine in a saucepan. Add the sugar, stirring until the mixture becomes slightly caramelized. Stir in the wholemeal flour and cook for 1 minute, stirring constantly. Remove the pan to the heat and cook, stirring constantly with a wooden spoon, for 2–3 minutes or until the sauce is thick and smooth. Pour the sauce into a sauceboat, arrange the lamb chops on a warmed serving dish on a bed of rice and pour sauce over them. Serve with bananas or sweetcorn and red pepper, lightly fried.

Braised Lamb with Peppers
   1 tablespoon oil
   2 lb shoulder lamb, boned and trimmed
   1 large onion, sliced
   1 large red pepper, de-seeded and sliced
   ½ pint hot water
   1 chicken cube, crushed
   Pepper
   6 oz potatoes, diced
   8 oz frozen peas

Method Heat oil in a large pan, add the lamb and brown it all over. Transfer the meat to a plate and add onion and pepper to pan. Stir fry until the vegetables begin to soften. Return joint to pan, placing it in the centre of the vegetables. Measure water, stir in the stock cube and seasoning and pour over the joint. Bring to boil, cover pan and simmer for 1 hour. Add potatoes and peas, bring back to simmering point, replace cover and continue cooking for a further 15 minutes. Transfer lamb to warm serving dish and serve it sliced, with the vegetables and stock gravy. Serves four.

Lamb with Yoghurt Sauce
   3 lamb steaks
   3 tablespoons clear honey
   3 tablespoons chopped mint
   1 tablespoon cider vinegar
   For the sauce
   ¼ pint natural yoghurt
   1 tablespoon clear honey
   1 tablespoon chopped parsley
   1 tablespoon chopped mint

Method Place meat in dish. Mix together the mint, honey and cider vinegar, pour it over the meat and leave to marinade for 2 hours. Cook under a hot grill for approximately 10 minutes each side, basting occasionally with the marinade liquid. Mix the sauce ingredients together and serve with the meat. A green salad is excellent with this dish.

Lamb Steaks with Pepper
  4 Tablespoons sunflower margarine
  1 Garlic clove, crushed
  Sea salt and pepper to taste
  1 lb lamb steaks, cut into strips
  4 tablespoons soya sauce
  2 teaspoons demerara sugar or honey
  6 oz bean sprouts
  2 green peppers, de-seeded and thinly sliced
  ½ tablespoon cornflour blended with 2 tablespoons water
  4 spring onions, sliced

Method Melt the margarine in large frying pan. Add the garlic, salt and pepper and stir fry for 30 seconds. Add the lamb strips and stir fry for 3 minutes. Increase the heat to high. Stir in the soya sauce and sugar or honey, cover and cook for 5 minutes. Uncover and stir in the bean sprouts and peppers. Cover again and simmer for 5 minutes. Stir in the cornflour until the mixture thickens. Put the mixture in a warmed serving dish, sprinkle it with spring onion and serve at once. Serves four.

Quick-fried Lamb Steaks with Vegetables
  ¼ cup sesame oil
  1 leek, separated and thinly sliced
  1 green pepper, de-seeded and thinly sliced
  2 oz button mushrooms, sliced
  4 oz bean sprouts

2 tablespoons soya sauce
2 lamb steaks, cut thinly

Method Heat half the oil in a large frying pan or wok. Add the leeks, peppers and mushrooms and stir fry for 3 minutes. Add the bean sprouts and soya sauce and stir fry for a further minute. Transfer the mixture to a warmed serving dish and keep hot. Put the remainder of the oil in the pan; when it is hot add the lamb steaks and cook for about 5 minutes each side, until they are cooked through. Arrange the steaks on top of the vegetables and serve at once. Serves two.

Lamb's Liver with Onions
1 oz sunflower margarine
2 tablespoons olive oil
3 onions, thinly sliced into rings
1½ lb lamb's liver, cut into strips
Sea salt and pepper to taste
Chopped parsley

Method Melt the margarine with the oil in a large, deep frying pan. Add the onions, reduce heat to low and simmer, stirring occasionally for 15 to 20 minutes, or until they are very soft. Meanwhile rub the liver strips with sea salt and pepper. Add the strips to the pan, raise the heat to moderate, and fry them for 4–6 minutes, turning occasionally, or until they are cooked through and tender. When all the liver has been cooked transfer the liver and onions to a warm serving dish and sprinkle with parsley. Serve at once.

Chicken Dishes

Chicken with Tarragon
8 tablespoons sunflower margarine
Sea salt and pepper

4 tablespoons chopped fresh tarragon
1 roasting chicken
6 tarragon sprigs

Method Pre-heat the oven to 190°C (375°F) (gas mark 5). Combine the margarine, seasoning and chopped tarragon and heat until they form a smooth paste. Stuff half the mixture inside the cavity of the chicken and fasten with a skewer. Put the chicken into a roasting pan, then spread the remaining butter mixture over the breast area. Put the pan into the oven and roast the chicken for 30 minutes, then turn it over and roast for another 30 minutes. Reduce the oven temperature to moderate 180°C (350°F)/gas mark 4. Turn the chicken onto its back and baste well with melted margarine. Roast for a further 30 minutes, basting well, or until chicken is cooked through. Remove from the oven and transfer chicken to a warmed serving dish. Pour the cooking juices over the chicken, garnish with tarragon sprigs and serve at once. Serves six.

Spanish Chicken
    ¼ cup olive oil
    4 lb chicken, cut into serving pieces
    2 medium onions, thinly sliced
    1 clove garlic, crushed
    1 large red pepper, de-seeded and chopped
    14 oz can artichoke hearts, drained
    2 cups chicken stock
    Sea salt and pepper to taste
    ¼ teaspoon cayenne pepper
    ½ teaspoon saffron threads soaked in tablespoon water
    16 stuffed olives, halved
    ½ tablespoon sunflower margarine and 1½ tablespoons
      flour, blended together

Method Pre-heat oven to moderate 180°C (350°F)/gas mark 4. Heat oil in large, deep frying pan. Add the chicken pieces and fry until they are evenly browned. Using tongs, transfer the pieces as they brown to a large flameproof casserole. Add the onions, garlic and pepper to the pan and fry until they are soft. Add the artichoke hearts and fry for a further 2 minutes. Pour over the stock and stir in the seasoning, cayenne and saffron. Bring to the boil, stirring occasionally. Pour the mixture over the chicken pieces. Put the casserole in the oven and cook for 1 hour, or until chicken pieces are cooked through and tender. Remove from oven and transfer chicken pieces to a warmed serving dish. Add olives to casserole and bring back to the boil. Stir in blended margarine and flour, until the sauce has thickened. Pour over chicken and serve.

Chicken Patrick
    1 tablespoon cider vinegar
    1 cupful diced cooked chicken
    ½ cupful sautéed mushrooms
    ¼ cupful diced canned pimento
    1 egg yolk
    3 tablespoons margarine
    3 tablespoons wholemeal flour
    1½ cups chicken stock
    Sea salt and pepper to taste

Method Melt the margarine in a saucepan, stir in and blend the wholemeal flour. Add the chicken stock slowly . When the mixture is smooth and boiling, add the chicken, mushrooms and pimento, reduce heat and add a lightly beaten egg yolk. Season with sea salt and pepper and add the cider vinegar. Serve on a bed of boiled rice.

Fried Chicken
    1 roasting chicken, jointed
    1 egg
    1 tablespoon water
    1 cup breadcrumbs

10 oz corn oil
½ teaspoon wholemeal flour seasoned with paprika, sea
  salt & peppered gravy
½ lb mushrooms
2 bananas
Lettuce

Method Pre-heat oven to 180°C (350°F)/gas mark 4. Heat
the oil in a deep saucepan. Toss the chicken pieces in
seasoned flour until well coated. Pile the breadcrumbs on a
plate. Beat the egg and water together and dip the chicken
pieces into the egg, then into the breadcrumbs, coating
them well. When the oil in the pan is boiling, add the
chicken pieces, two or three at a time, and fry until they are
golden brown all over. When the pieces have all been fried
for about 5 minutes, place them in a baking tin with ½ pint
melted margarine and cook in the oven until tender. Allow
about 1 ½ hours cooking time. When cooked, place the
pieces on a serving dish. Serve them garnished with fried
mushrooms and bananas, and shredded lettuce.

Chicken and Nut Galantine
  1 medium-sized roasting chicken
  1 pint water
  A pinch of sea salt
  Freshly ground black pepper
  4 oz chopped nuts
  2 oz soft brown breadcrumbs
  2 eggs, beaten
  ⅔ cup chicken stock

Method Cut all the meat from the chicken and set aside.
Put the bones and giblets in a saucepan with the water and
salt and pepper to taste. Cover the pan and simmer for 1
hour. Mince the chicken with the meat from the giblets and
add the nuts and breadcrumbs. Stir in the eggs and chicken
stock and add salt and pepper to taste. Press the mixture

into a well-greased 2lb loaf tin and cover with greased foil. Stand in a roasting tin containing a little cold water. Place in a pre-heated moderate oven, 180°C (350°F)/gas mark 4, and cook for 1¼–1½ hours. Leave to cool. Serve cold with salad or for picnics or packed lunches.

Normandy Chicken
  1 tablespoon corn oil
  ½ cup sunflower margarine
  3 lb chicken, cut into portions
  2 shallots, finely chopped
  1 oz wholemeal flour
  2 cups cider vinegar
  ½ cup chicken stock
  ½ teaspoon dried sage
  ¼ teaspoon dried thyme
  Sea salt
  Freshly ground black pepper
  1 lb dessert apples, peeled, cored and thickly sliced

Method Heat the oil and half the margarine in a frying pan and fry the chicken portions until golden brown all over. Remove the chicken portions from the pan and transfer to a casserole. Fry the shallots in the fat remaining in the pan, then sprinkle in the flour and cook, stirring constantly, until light brown. Gradually stir in the cider vinegar, stock and herbs and bring to the boil, stirring constantly. Cook until the sauce has thickened, season to taste with sea salt and pepper and pour over the chicken. Cover the casserole, place in a pre-heated oven, 180°C (350°F)/gas mark 4, and cook for 1 hour or until the chicken is just tender. Meanwhile melt the remaining margarine in a pan and cook the apple slices for about 2 minutes, stirring occasionally until golden brown. Spoon the apples over the chicken, taste and adjust seasoning. Serves six.

Chicken with Mushroom Sauce
  4 chicken pieces
  ½ teaspoon chopped fresh marjoram or rosemary
  1 teaspoon sea salt
  A pinch of freshly ground black pepper
  1 teaspoon chopped fresh chives
  ⅓ cup cider vinegar
  3 tablespoons margarine
  ¼ cup wholemeal flour
  1 ¼ cups skimmed milk
  1 ½ cups sliced mushrooms

Method Put the chicken in a deep casserole large enough to hold the joints in a single layer. Sprinkle with herbs, salt and pepper to taste, chives and cider vinegar. Dot with small knobs of margarine. Cut the mushrooms into small pieces. Cover with foil or a lid. Place in a pre-heated oven, 180°C (350°F)/gas mark 4, and bake for 45 minutes. Melt the remaining margarine in a saucepan and stir in the flour. Cook, stirring, for 1 minute. Gradually add the milk, stirring constantly, and bring to the boil. Stir in the juices from the chicken and the mushrooms. Simmer for 2 minutes. Taste and adjust the seasoning. Serves four.

Chicken with Prunes
  ⅔ cup prunes, soaked
  5 onions, 1 sliced and 4 quartered
  1 bay leaf
  6 peppercorns
  1 cup cider vinegar
  4 chicken pieces
  2 tablespoons olive oil
  2 tablespoons sunflower margarine
  ¼ cup wholemeal flour
  ⅔ cup chicken stock
  ½ teaspoon sea salt
  Freshly ground black pepper

Method Put the prunes in a saucepan with the sliced onion, bay leaf, peppercorns and cider vinegar. Bring slowly to boil, then allow to cool. Add the chicken joints. Turn into a bowl, cover and leave to marinate overnight or for several hours in the refrigerator. Strain off the marinade and set aside. Stone the prunes. Fry the chicken quickly in oil and margarine until golden brown. Remove the onions from the pan. Blend the flour with the fat remaining in the pan and gradually add the marinade, stirring constantly. Bring to the boil, stirring. Add the stock, sea salt and pepper and stir well. Return the chicken, quartered onions and prunes to the pan. Cover and simmer for 45 minutes or until the chicken is tender. Taste and adjust the seasoning. Serves four.

Country Chicken and Mushroom Pie

1 roasting chicken
2 onions, peeled
2 carrots, roughly chopped
6 black peppercorns
1 bouquet garni
Sea salt
¼ cup sunflower margarine
2 cups thinly-sliced mushrooms
¼ cup wholemeal flour
½ cup natural yoghurt
1 teaspoon chopped fresh tarragon
Freshly ground black pepper
For the piecrust
½ lb pastry
1 egg, beaten

Method Put the chicken in a large saucepan with a quartered onion, the carrots, peppercorns, bouquet garni, and sea salt to taste. Barely cover the chicken with water and bring to the boil. Lower the heat, cover and simmer gently for an hour or until the chicken is tender. Remove the pan from the heat and leave the chicken to cool in the cooking liquid. Take the chicken out of the pan, strain and reserve the liquid. Take the chicken meat from the bones and cut into bite-sized pieces, discarding any skin. Chop the remaining onion finely and fry it gently in margarine until soft and golden. Add the mushrooms and fry for another 2 minutes. Sprinkle in the flour and cook for 1 minute. Stir $\frac{2}{3}$ cup of reserved cooking liquid into the natural yoghurt. Add this to the pan and bring slowly to the boil, stirring, then simmer for 2 minutes, stirring constantly until the sauce thickens. Remove the pan from the heat and add the tarragon, sea salt and pepper to taste. Stir the chicken pieces into the sauce and transfer to a pie dish. Put a pie funnel at the centre of the pie dish. Roll out the pastry on a floured surface. Dampen the rim. Cover the filling with the pastry, pressing down firmly to seal. Trim the edges with a sharp knife and use the trimmings to decorate the top of the pie. Brush the pastry with beaten egg. Stand the pie dish on a pre-heated baking sheet, place in a pre-heated oven, 200°C (400°F)/gas mark 6, and bake for 30 minutes or until the pie is heated through and bubbling and the pastry is golden brown. Serve hot with a green vegetable.

Chicken and Mushroom Casserole
    3 lb chicken, cut into pieces
    2 tablespoons sunflower margarine
    $\frac{3}{4}$ lb onions, peeled and chopped
    4 celery stalks, cut into pieces
    $\frac{1}{4}$ cup wholemeal flour
    1 $\frac{1}{4}$ pints chicken stock
    1 bouquet garni
    Sea salt
    Freshly ground black pepper
    1 cup button mushrooms

Method Fry the chicken in the margarine until golden brown all over, then transfer to casserole dish. Cook onions and celery in the fat remaining in the pan for about 10 minutes, then stir in the flour and cook for 1 minute. Gradually add the stock and bring to the boil, stirring constantly. Add the bouquet garni, season with sea salt and pepper to taste and pour the sauce over the chicken. Cover and place in a pre-heated moderate oven, 180°C (350°F)/ gas mark 4, and cook for 45 minutes. Add the mushrooms and cook for a further 15 minutes. Remove the bouquet garni. Taste and adjust the seasoning. Serve with boiled rice, peas and sweet corn. Serves four.

Dessert Recipes

Apple Crumble
1 lb baking apples, peeled, cored and thinly sliced
½–⅔ cup Barbados sugar
For the crumble topping
1½ cups self-raising wholemeal flour
⅓ cup sunflower margarine
⅓ cup Barbados sugar
A pinch of ground cinnamon

Method Place fruit in pie dish, layering with sugar to taste. To make topping, sift the flour into a bowl, rub in the margarine until the mixture resembles breadcrumbs, then stir in the sugar and cinammon. Sprinkle the crumble evenly over the fruit, smooth the top and press down lightly. Place in a pre-heated oven, 210°C (425°F)/gas mark 7, and bake for 20 minutes, then reduce the temperature to moderately hot, 190°C (375°F)/gas mark 5, and cook for a further 45 minutes. Serves four.

Mixed Fruit Pudding
1 cup self-raising wholemeal flour
A pinch of sea salt
1 teaspoon baking powder
½ teaspoon mixed spice

½ teaspoon ground cinnamon
⅔ cup demerara sugar
2 cups fresh breadcrumbs
⅓ cup raisins
½ cup currants
½ cup seedless white raisins
2 medium eggs, beaten
½ cup skimmed milk

Method Sift the flour, salt, baking powder, mixed spice and cinnamon together into a bowl and stir in the sugar, breadcrumbs and dried fruit. Stir in the beaten egg and enough milk to give a soft consistency. Spoon the mixture into a pudding basin rubbed with sunflower margarine. Cover with foil, making a pleat in the centre to allow for expansion. Secure the foil around the rim of the basin with string. Stand in a saucepan with boiling water to one-third the depth of the basin and steam for 2½ hours, topping up with boiling water when necessary. Serves four or six.

Almond and Brown Sugar Flan
For the pastry
2 cups wholemeal flour
½ teaspoon sea salt
½ cup sunflower margarine
1–2 tablespoons water
For the filling
½ cup sunflower margarine
⅔ cup demerara sugar
1 large egg, beaten
½ cup finely-chopped, blanched almonds
1 cup self-raising wholemeal flour sifted with ½ teaspoon cinnamon
1 tablespoon skimmed milk
1 tablespoon seedless white raisins

Method To make pastry, sift the flour and salt together into a bowl then rub in the margarine until the mixture resembles fine breadcrumbs. Stir in enough water to make a firm dough. Knead the dough lightly on a floured surface for 1 minute. Wrap in foil and leave to chill in the refrigerator for 30 minutes. Roll out the dough on a floured surface and use to line an 8-inch flan tin. To make the filling, place the margarine and sugar in a bowl and beat until the mixture is light and fluffy. Beat in the eggs and almonds a little at a time, then fold in the sifted flour and cinnamon alternately with the skimmed milk. Stir in the seedless white raisins and turn the mixture into the pastry-lined flan tin, smoothing the top with a knife. Place in a pre-heated, hot oven 210°C (425°F)/gas mark 7, and bake for 15 minutes, then reduce the temperature to moderate, 190°C (375°F)/gas mark 5, and bake for a further 25 minutes or until browned. Remove the flan from the oven and leave to cool.

Cinnamon Apple Pancakes
  For the batter
  1 cup wholemeal flour
  A pinch of sea salt
  1 egg
  1 tablespoon corn oil
  1 ¼ cups skimmed milk
  Corn oil for frying
  For the filling
  4 large baking apples, peeled, cored and sliced
  A pinch of ground cinnamon
  1 cup raw brown sugar
  ½ cup sunflower margarine

Method To make the batter, sift the flour and sea salt into a bowl. Blend in the egg, corn oil and enough skimmed milk to make a fairly thin batter. Heat a little oil in a frying pan. Drop 2 tablespoons of batter into the centre of the pan and tilt and rotate to spread it. Cook for 1 minute. Turn the pancake over and cook the other side for 1 minute. Turn the pancake out of the pan and make nine or ten more in the same way. Leave to cool. For the filling put the apples, cinnamon, sugar and margarine in a saucepan and simmer gently for about 20 minutes or until the apple is tender, stirring occasionally. Roll some of the filling in each pancake and fry the pancake rolls in margarine over moderate heat until they are golden brown all over. Pile on a warm serving dish and sprinkle with a mixture of sugar and cinnamon. Serve with low-fat ice cream. Serves five or six.

Apple and Almond Jelly
  2 large, sweet raw apples
  ¼ lb ground almonds
  ¾ oz gelatine
  ½ pint water
  ½ pint apple juice
  1 tablespoon thick honey

Method Grate the apples and mix with the almonds. Dissolve the gelatine in ½ pint water and stir in the honey and apple juice. Put the apple mixture into a large mould and pour in the liquid. Allow to set, turn out and serve with low-fat ice cream.

Plain Sponge
  ¼ lb wholemeal flour, sieved
  ¼ lb brown sugar
  3 oz sunflower margarine
  1 tablespoon milk
  2 eggs

Method Cream margarine and sugar, add the eggs one at a time and beat thoroughly. Fold in the sieved flour. Add milk if necessary, the mixture should be fairly stiff. Divide into 7-inch sandwich tins and bake at 180°C (350°F)/ gas mark 4, for 15–20 minutes. Turn on to cake rack to cool or serve hot with custard made with skimmed or powdered milk.

For a healthy finish to a meal, I don't think there is anything to beat a fresh fruit salad. A variety of fruits (except citrus or any acid fruit) can be cut into small chunks and topped with a little low-fat ice cream.

6

The Clinic

Positive thinking is the essence of all healing. Many patients have said to me that they came to my clinic full of
miseries – and went away full of hope. Hopeful that they
are going to feel better in a short time and hopeful that
eventually they will get rid of their arthritis. Faith in
oneself is the essence of joyful living – when one has faith,
there is no room for worry. Worry is the downfall of all who
can't fight it – so I say, don't try to fight it. Instead adopt a
positive mental attitude and when waking each morning,
thank God for allowing you to wake up, and for giving you
the opportunity to enjoy the beautiful new day that he has
ordained for you, think of others and how you can help
them, and it's surprising the sense of well-being and satis-
faction that one derives from a kind thought, word or deed,
projected in the direction of our fellow man.

Always think pleasant and happy thoughts as you lay
your head on your pillow, because you shape and build
your character and willpower while you are asleep. If your
dominant thought when you fall asleep is cheerful and
happy, you will wake up cheerful, strong and resolute to
begin another day. Always aim high and don't be content
with pettiness, and above all watch a 'don't care' frame of
mind. Forget the past, that is gone – look to a bright, happy
and successful future. It is what you are capable of doing
now that matters, and you are capable of big things if you
will put your shoulder to the wheel and push with all your
might.

Don't fear, don't fret, don't anticipate evil, don't fear
anything for there is nothing to fear, fret or worry about.
Hold your head high, look the world in the face, fight the
good fight and victory will be yours.

I find that most people that I see at the clinic think

negatively, and I am fully convinced that this negative thinking destroys them. 'There is no cure – you must learn to live with it' – what negative thinking, and what a death sentence! That sentence was pronounced on me, and to this day I believe that if I didn't have a husband and a large family to look after, I might not have had the willpower to fight the good fight and rid myself of that painful body that was the result of wrong diet. However, I thank the Lord that he gave me so many reasons to explore every channel for the promotion of good health, and a pain-free busy life.

Miss K., an eighteen-year-old college student, came to my clinic. In the course of conversation I asked her what she intended to do when she finished her education. She said: 'I did hope to be a chemist, Nurse Hills, but they [the doctors] told me they can do nothing for my arthritis, so I expect I shall end up a spinster in a wheelchair.' It has taken me a long time and several visits to inject positive thought into that girl's mind, and now she has reduced her drugs to a minimum and I had such a joyful call from her brother a couple of weeks ago to say she was playing badminton. Before she came to me she had tremendous difficulty dressing herself and experienced very severe pain in her feet when she walked.

Miss T., a retired secretary, was diagnosed as having arthritis of the elbows and knees a few months before she retired. Her doctor told her that there is no cure. She rang me in desperation, saying she had no intention of spending her retirement indoors in pain and could I do anything. I made an appointment for her on 23 June; by the 10 August she was feeling a lot better, by 14 October she was getting very little pain and the swellings were disappearing. By 10 December there was no pain and no swelling and she was looking the picture of health. On the 4 May 1984 she was examined by her doctor and found clear of arthritis.

Mr T., aged sixty, had very bad arthritis in both knees. He came to the clinic on 21 October 1983, walking painfully with the help of two sticks. He was currently taking two drugs for his arthritis; he had high blood pressure. He undertook to follow my treatment religiously every day – and by 6 February, he was totally free of any discomfort and had returned to a full-time job. That complete transformation had come about in the course of less than four months – again, he couldn't believe his good luck.

Then there was Mrs W. – she had suffered badly with arthritis for about seven years. Her hands were severely deformed and she had lost all power. She came to the clinic on 6 June 1983. She stuck rigidly to the diet and treatment and by October she had regained the use of her hands; the power had come back to the extent that she could now open a tin of dog food with an old-fashioned opener, where before she couldn't even pick up the tin.

Miss C., a retired teacher, came to see me on 11 November 1983. She had had arthritis for twelve years – she was seventy years of age. Her arthritis was getting worse and she was becoming extremely hard to live with. She was very overweight and was on drugs. She came for a second appointment on the 11 January 1984. She had lost a stone in weight on the diet she had been prescribed and this in turn had relieved the pressure on her aching knees; she was feeling better than she had felt for years and had developed a positive, happy outlook. She has now lost another three pounds and her pains are subsiding a lot. She is confident that eventually she is going to be well, and with that air of confidence she can only get better as the days go by.

My patients become my friends, I take a personal interest in each and every one of them. To treat a patient properly one has to ascertain an over-all picture of the patient's life style, his or her worries and frustrations, because these play an important part in the attitude of a patient towards the illness.

Very often a patient will come to my clinic, having lost a spouse recently; he will tell me he is living alone and trying to adjust to life without his partner. He says his arthritis has got so much worse since his partner passed away. He can see himself ending up in a wheelchair with nobody to look after him, and he projects a picture of hopelessness. I try to tell this patient that there is nothing to fear in life except fear. I ask him to cast out fear and look forward with hope; not just a vague hope in the mind, but hope throbbing as a life force in the heart. I say that death does not divide, there is no need to fear separation and death can never separate souls who love. It is very comforting to realize that however difficult you find life, if you accept your circumstances graciously and thankfully you will press forward rekindled by the fires of hope and know that in the end all will be well.

Usually when somebody falls sick something is lacking, and there is an imbalance in the patient's soul. Sometimes it is very difficult to ascertain the reasons for that imbalance, sometimes it is never ascertained, but with most people, as I gain their confidence, little by little the story unfolds and gradually I can see the reason, or reasons, for their state of ill-health.

I believe in helping my patients to help themselves, and as every healer knows, true healing begins with the spirit. As soon as the spirit practises pure thinking, pure living and pure action, it experiences a sense of well-being not previously known and starts to live harmoniously within itself. The aches, pains and frustrations recede into the background and a sense of faith in himself, coupled with a hopeful attitude, and kindness towards his fellow man replaces them. The power of positive thinking can bring forth beauty and harmony in a patient's life and by good, constructive ideas he can help to bring about that which is desirable and good.

Quite often I receive letters or phone calls of gratitude from my patients; it is encouraging to me to know that yet another of my patients is free of pain and does not require my services any longer. I give thanks to God and feel very humble and grateful that I have once again been instrumental in relieving another's pain and enabling that person to lead a pain-free, balanced, useful life.

Perhaps the following extract from a patient's letter will encourage the reader not to lose heart and set about self-help, as this patient has done:

> I am filled with gratitude for the help you gave me, getting me to walk like a human being again. I contacted you in June 1983. What a wreck I was, crying, cringing, a mess of a woman, in complete despair – you changed all that. I stuck to your diet and treatment religiously, now, here I am, decorating the house, and gardening and trimming my poodle. I am back in the stream of life, not 'up the creek' as I surely thought I was.

The above patient was brought to my clinic on 18 June 1983. She could not sit on a chair and had been lying on her back for five months, under medical care. She had to lie on the floor on an eiderdown while I examined her. She had lost a lot of weight and was very confused. I knelt on the floor beside her and put my hands on her back asking if that was where the trouble was. She said, 'Yes, that's it. Please keep your hands there, don't take them away, they are very hot'. I realized that my hands were being used to bring warmth and comfort to that patient and I prayed that the pain would go. When I stood up after fifteen minutes, the pain had gone and the patient stood up straight for the first time in five months and cried tears of joy, saying 'I'm healed'. She walked out to the car. I phoned her on Monday, 20 June at 9 am to confirm the healing, she reported that she had been feeling fantastic since Saturday. She had made early morning tea and hoovered through the house. For the past eleven months she has followed the treatment and diet I set out for her; now she has put on weight and is doing all the things she wants to do – or as she puts it, she is 'back in the stream of life'. I do not profess to be a spiritual healer, although I do believe wholeheartedly in spiritual healing – but something happened that

Saturday afternoon in June 1983 that both my patient and I will never cease to give thanks for.

Miss B. had arthritis for years and was getting steadily worse, I saw her on the 28 January 1984. She was very depressed. On the second appointment which was on 15 March 1984 she had developed a totally different outlook. She said she 'felt wonderful' and could get up and down stairs much better than before. She said she couldn't believe the improvement.

Mr M. came to see me in August 1982. He was thirty-four years old and had four children; he had lost his job and his wife was at her wits' end because she had an ailing husband and four children to look after. He started the diet and treatment I prescribed for him and the following March he wrote to me to say that he had been to the hospital for X-rays and blood tests, and was told there was no arthritis left in his body. He had put on weight, had got his job back and had been promoted, and all in a matter of six months. It is widely believed that nothing in this world happens without purpose, and I very often think that the fact that I had to suffer the pain of arthritis for sixteen years was arranged on purpose so that I can relate now to my patients, and realize at first hand the intensity of their pains.

On 12 June 1982 an article appeared in the *Coventry Evening Telegraph*. It read as follows: 'Nobody knows what causes arthritis, there is no cure for it, the Coventry Council are spending X amounts of money on research and in three years they hope to come up with a cure.' Needless to say, they are now two years on and they still haven't found a cure and, in my opinion, never will while they look to drugs for the answer. As I have said and proved, the cure lies in our own efforts to rid our bodies of uric acid to keep to an acid-free diet and partake of the vitamins and minerals necessary to return to a state of health.

When I read that article I had a compulsion to pick up my pen and write to the paper of my experience. When they got my letter, they telephoned me to ask for my photograph, which I reluctantly allowed them to take – I am not particularly proud of my figure, as the bearing of eight children and the passage of the years have not exactly enhanced it. However, I was duly photographed and my story printed in the paper and then the dilemma began. My phone never stopped ringing. As soon as I answered one call there was another arthritis sufferer on the line. I had to take the phone off the hook, I could get no peace and could not get through my work.

During the two remaining weeks in June, over 4,000 letters cascaded through my door; the postman asked if he could leave them in bundles on the doorstep. I had treatment leaflets printed and sent to each person who wrote, and between June and September I sent treatment leaflets to people in practically every country in the world. I made appointments at my home, charging £5 a time which helped to cover printing costs (and any left over I gave to charity). And so my clinic began; it is now thriving and going from strength to strength.

In the past six months I have realized that the volume of suffering is so great that I cannot possibly hope to reach enough people on a one-to-one basis at the clinic, so I now book hotel rooms at weekends when the clinic is closed, and go out amongst the people in various parts of the Midlands, telling them how to relieve their pains the natural way. Sometimes the numbers waiting to hear the talks are so great that as soon as I finish one talk, I have to start another; at one particular hotel they kept ringing up to see if there was a third talk.

Typical of the press reports following the talks is this one:

Phone Calls Galore Over Arthritis Talk – Arthritis sufferers searching for a cure have besieged a hotel near Stourbridge which staged a talk on natural methods of beating the painful condition. Now, the nurse who gave the talk has appealed for people to get in touch with her instead of bombarding the Stewponey Hotel at Stourton with phone calls. More than 200 people turned up at the talk given by Nurse Margaret Hills on Saturday and an extra session had to be put on for dozens of others who had to be turned away.

Since the talk was reported in the Wolverhampton & Stourbridge press hundreds of people had phoned the hotel asking for more information about my methods of treating arthritis. The hotel manager told me, 'The response has been unbelievable – the phone has not stopped ringing. I have never realized that there was so much concern about arthritis. We must have had more than 1,000 calls since the talk was reported.'

Newspapers connected with my talks are reporting in a similar manner in various parts of the Midlands. It has made me realize that the amount of suffering is astronomical. It is widespread, in every country of the world.

This realization resulted in my decision to adopt a system of treatment by post, as all arthritics suffer in much the same way, to a greater or lesser degree. The system seems to be working extremely well; holistic treatment is carried out as far as is possible.

I hope and pray that the publication of this book will help to alleviate at least some of the pain and suffering, and bring hope to so many who have heard those hopeless words 'there is no cure – you must learn to live with it'. I say, be hopeful; now you know there is a cure and you do not have to learn to live with it, but remember, perseverance is the answer.

The treatment is constantly being reviewed, and anyone wishing latest information should write enclosing a stamped self-addressed envelope to:

The Margaret Hills Clinic, 4 Stoneleigh Road, Gibbet Hill, Coventry CV4 7AD.

I hope that by now the reader will have adopted a

positive attitude of mind towards his or her illness and I should like everyone to remember the old adage – 'Whatever the mind of man can believe and perceive, it can achieve'.

I thank you for reading this book and hope you will benefit from it. May I also thank my many patients who have helped me and taught me so much along the way.

Good luck and God bless you all.

Index

Neuritis 44, 45
Nutrition 12, 16, 21, 28,
36, 40–1, 42, 49–51

Obesity 23, 51
Optimism 20, *see also*
  Positive thinking
Osteo-arthritis 2, 5
Osteomalacia 46

Pain 5, 6, 11, 19, 27, 33
Pernicious anaemia 45
Phosphoric acid 29, 46
Pollen 27
Porridge 55–6, 63
Positive thinking 20, 34,
  36, 59, 93–101
Potassium 29, 30
Pruritis 11
Psoriasis 30

Quinsy 9

Recipes for arthritis
  sufferers
  breakfast 63–9
  grilled fish 69–75
  meat 75–80
  desserts 88–92
Rickets 46, 49
Rheumatoid arthritis 1, 3,
  5
Royal College of
  Physicians 17

Salt, in diet 36, 53
Sciatica 11
Self-help 14, *see also*
  Positive thinking
Shingles 9
Smoking 28, 35, 36, 42
Solar plexus 9
'Spontaneous
  remission' 13
St Vitus's Dance 9
Stress 27, 28, 40
  avoidance of 34–6
Sugar, refined 8, 50–1
Synovial membrane 6

Tannic acid 40, 61, 62
Toxic acids 8, 15, 18, 20,
  21, 43

Ulcers 29–30, 61, 62
Uric acid 5, 8, 15, 19, 23,
  29, 33, 58

Vertigo 9
Vitamins 19, 21, 26, 27–8,
  37, 40, 42–52, 53, 55, 58
Vomiting 17

Well-being, feelings of 6,
  40, 50, 57, 93, 96
Wholefoods 42, 50–2, 54
Worry 93

Xerophthalmia 44
X-rays 98